"In *The Milltown Boys at Sixty*, the indefatigable masterclass in ethnography that offers a nuanced ⁝ ... ..., ... it is like to grow up and old(er) in lives that began on a social housing estate. Williamson does a superb job of allowing some of the 'The Boys', whom he first met when they were 13 or 14 and who are now 60, reflect back across the years on lives lived mostly on the margins, whilst offering social commentary on the institutions - labour market, criminal justice services, and social and health services - that repeatedly failed many of them, then and now. The inclusion of themes such as who has succeeded and what success means, who counts as family, the role of belief systems and identity, and the far-reaching effects of mental health struggles make this account relevant and timely. A story of young lives - their origins and destinations - told across nearly fifty years is rare, but then so is Howard Williamson — a reflective and compassionate youth worker, youth policy expert and youth sociologist who has spent his entire career in the service of young people. *The Milltown Boys at Sixty* challenges us to change our approach from youth studies to life histories, our academic gaze from distant to intimate, and our analysis from a single lens to that of a kaleidoscope. Congratulations Howard, we are very proud of you!"

—**Sharlene Swartz**, *President, Sociology of Youth Research Committee, International Sociological Association, Professor of Philosophy, University of Fort Hare, South Africa*

"With this book Howard Williamson returns to the story of the 'Milltown Boys' as they reach the age of 60. First met as teenagers, that Prof Williamson has retained close contact with these men over such an extended period is a very rare, perhaps unique sociological achievement. The twists and turns of the lives of 'the Boys' — family lives and friendships, encounters with crime and the criminal justice system, with jobs and unemployment, experiences of ageing and bereavement - are recounted with sensitivity, care and humour. This is not a typical academic book — not least because it is extraordinarily engaging! It rings with ethnographic truth. It should be relevant to a range of university courses in sociology, criminology, youth studies, youth work and research methodology. I can imagine students reading this book with great enthusiasm."

—**Robert MacDonald**, *Co-editor in Chief, Journal of Youth Studies, Professor of Education and Social Justice, University of Huddersfield, United Kingdom*

"*The Milltown Boys at Sixty* studies the same group of boys and men for a period of nearly 50 years. This extensive qualitative longitudinal study examines themes such as growing up, working, maintaining friendships, getting older and even facing the inevitable brevity of human lives. Professor Williamson's reflections on research ethics and building relations with the people he studies are distinctive and immensely interesting. The book looks at life courses from the inside, and connects them to relevant themes in youth sociology without colonising the richness of the everyday with too much theory. The book offers narratives that are simultaneously a contribution to social science and evocative examples of long lives well lived, filled with beauty and dignity."

"Understanding people's lives requires genuine empathy with others, sociological sense and sensitivity, and methodological imagination. It takes wit and it takes time. This book, in itself an autobiographical narrative account of how 'strange fascinations' change over time, is an example of these qualities. It is a reminder of the social and sociological reflexivity and honesty that comes with studying youth and beyond. This third act of the 'Milltown Boys' is an inspired and inspirational piece of sociological storytelling."

"Howard Williamson has done it again! Professor Williamson is a masterful storyteller, and has once again written a fascinating page-turner. This time he has produced a one of a kind longitudinal ethnography, spanning the lives of 'the Boys' over five decades, a group of socially disadvantaged (young) men with whom he became closely acquainted in his own youth. Williamson's attention to detail in his close personal relationships with his respondents comes out on every page. Written in a conversational style, he shows how his own biography is intertwined with 'the Boys' he studied for those five decades, as his life course paralleled—but contrasted—their varied life courses. Indeed, the detailed narrative of the ethnographer's experiences is as interesting as the personal narratives he has documented from his respondents. This third edition of *The Milltown Boys* is must-read for youth studies researchers, but also scholars from many disciplines, especially those studying offenders—young and old alike—including sociology, social work, criminology, psychology, and psychiatry."

"H, it's fantastic; it brought it all back. You put yourself in there - that's what you had to do. You weren't like that Roundhouse bloke, who couldn't go back. It was all about trust, H, trust - that's why we let you in in the first place, H, we trusted you. And we still do. That's the thing, H, it was never about money; we knew you didn't care about money, we knew you were interested in us. I cried, H, I laughed, it brought back so much. You've got it all in there. It's special, H. I bet there's nothing quite like it. Because nobody's done it before. Not stuck around with Boys like us for as long as you have…"

"It's great, H. I've really enjoyed reading it. I don't like everything you've said about me, but there you are – warts and all! And you're in it, like you should be. We wanted you to be more like one of the Boys, more included, more visible. And that's what you've done, H, that's what you've done."

THE MILLTOWN BOYS AT SIXTY

The Milltown Boys at Sixty is a story like no other, giving both an insider and an outsider view of the 'Milltown Boys', exploring the nature of an ethnographic relationship based on research about their experiences of the criminal justice system.

A group classically labelled as delinquents, drug-takers and drop-outs, the Boys were also, in many different ways, fathers, friends and family men, differentially immersed in the labour market, in very different family relationships and now very differently connected to criminal activity. Williamson has written books capturing their experiences over the 50 years of his continued association with them: about their teenage years; and 20 years later, in middle age. This book is about them as they pass the age of 60, providing a personal account of the relationship between Williamson and the Boys, and the distinctive – perhaps even controversial – research methodology that enabled the mapping of their lives. It provides a unique and detailed insight into the ways in which the lives of the Milltown Boys that started with such shared beginnings have unfolded in so many diverse and fascinating ways.

These accounts will be of interest to the lay reader curious about the way others have managed (or failed to manage) their lives, the professional who works with those living, often struggling, on the wrong side of the tracks, and the academic researching and teaching about social exclusion, substance misuse, criminal justice transitions and the life course.

Howard Williamson is Professor of European Youth Policy at the University of South Wales. His academic work has focused on youth, social exclusion and public policy. He recently completed the editing of a seven-volume *History of Youth Work in Europe*, published by the Council of Europe.

THE MILLTOWN BOYS AT SIXTY

The Origins and Destinations of Young Men from a Poor Neighbourhood

Howard Williamson

Luke + Lucy,
wishing you all the
very best with the
project. When it's
done, I look forward
to the housewarming
and you may then
have time to read
this book!

Howard.

30. 5. 21

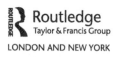
Routledge
Taylor & Francis Group

LONDON AND NEW YORK

First published 2021
by Routledge
2 Park Square, Milton Park, Abingdon, Oxon OX14 4RN

and by Routledge
52 Vanderbilt Avenue, New York, NY 10017

Routledge is an imprint of the Taylor & Francis Group, an informa business

British Library Cataloguing-in-Publication Data
A catalogue record for this book is available from the British Library

Library of Congress Cataloging-in-Publication Data
Names: Williamson, Howard, author.
Title: The Milltown boys at sixty : the origins and destinations of young
men from a poor neighbourhood / Howard Williamson.
Description: Abingdon, Oxon ; New York, NY : Routledge, 2021. |
Includes bibliographical references and index.
Identifiers: LCCN 2020054471 (print) | LCCN 2020054472 (ebook) |
ISBN 9780367725143 (hbk) | ISBN 9780367725228 (pbk) |
ISBN 9781003155102 (ebk)
Subjects: LCSH: Poor–Great Britain–Longitudinal studies. |
Poor men–Great Britain–Case studies.
Classification: LCC HC260.P6 W488 2021 (print) |
LCC HC260.P6 (ebook) | DDC 305.5/6909429–dc23
LC record available at https://lccn.loc.gov/2020054471
LC ebook record available at https://lccn.loc.gov/2020054472

ISBN: 978-0-367-72514-3 (hbk)
ISBN: 978-0-367-72522-8 (pbk)
ISBN: 978-1-003-15510-2 (ebk)

Typeset in Bembo
by Newgen Publishing UK

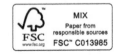

Printed in the United Kingdom
by Henry Ling Limited

Dedicated to 'Adrian', Gary's son
(1993–2017)
It was his death that enabled this book to come to life.

Edinburgh's International Award for Young People, and a board member of the European Forum Alpbach Foundation.

He writes prolifically, publishing not only academic books and journal articles but also columns for magazines and newspapers. His most recent work has been synthesising ideas about youth policy in Europe, co-editing the seven volumes of the *History of Youth Work in Europe*, and co-authoring a revised *Youth Policy Manual* for the EU–Council of Europe youth partnership.

Since 2002, he has been Organisational Secretary of the International Sociological Association Research Committee 34, the global network for the sociology of youth. He was also chair of the European Network of Youth Research Correspondents until 2008.

In his spare time, he rides horses and motorbikes, plays the guitar and harmonica, and is a football coach and qualified referee, and Safeguarding Officer for Pontypridd Town Association Football Club.

In 2002, he was appointed a Commander of the Order of the British Empire (CBE), for services to young people, and in 2016, he was appointed a Commander of the Royal Victorian Order (CVO). In 2019, he was presented with an 'Outstanding Contribution to Youth Work' Youth Work Excellence Award by the First Minister of Wales.

PREFACE

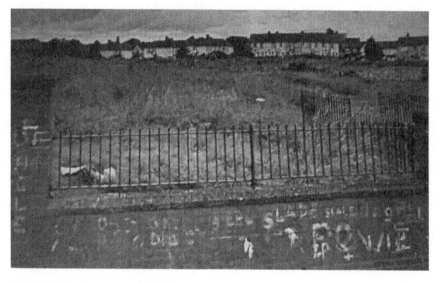

PHOTO 1 Graffiti on a wall in Milltown

"You're very privileged to have known us!" (Tony)
"Life goes on. We're still here to tell the story" (Mark)
"Other than getting older, not a lot has changed" (Kelvin)

A shot of Milltown taken sometime in the 2010s in front of some wasteland – the graffiti in the foreground was sprayed by some of the Boys in the 1970s!

I moved to Milltown and met the 'Milltown Boys' in the summer of 1973. They were 13 or 14 years old. I spent a great deal of time with them – at first, for a couple of years, volunteering in the 'youth club' at the recreation ground (it was officially an adventure playground), then subsequently, for the next three years, hanging around on the streets and in the woods, going to football matches, attending court and visiting them in various custodial institutions. I wrote a book about those five years of growing up on the estate: Five Years. After that, I lost contact with many, though not all, of the Boys. I stayed in touch with the central core of my contacts – particularly Danny, Marty, Jerry, Ted and, to a lesser extent, Pete. Twenty years later, for various reasons, I decided to try to find them again and see how their lives had unfolded. Of 67 names on a list I drew up, with Danny's help, in 1999 I learned that seven of the Boys were dead, none from natural causes. I thought I would try to interview half of the 60 who remained. By the end of 2000, I had interviewed 30 of the Boys. The Milltown Boys Revisited *was published in 2004. By 2008, I had shaken hands with 47 of those 60 men.*

As 2020 approached, having had sporadic engagement with a few of the Boys throughout that time, and having deliberated for at least six years as to whether or not to embark on 'further research', I thought I might just try to renew contact with at least some of them (perhaps a dozen or so), through social media and personal communication. This book is the result, perhaps less of an academic account than I might have produced and more of a personal account of an interesting relationship over a lifetime – between the working-class Milltown Boys and a middle-class man who stumbled upon them purely by chance when he was a university student. It is based on one 'context setting' interview with one of the more reflective of the Boys who had not been included in my studies in the past and 12 in-depth online interviews, supplemented by word-of-mouth information, material from phone calls and voicemails, Messenger exchanges and text messages, Facebook material, internet blogs and WhatsApp encounters.

ACKNOWLEDGEMENTS

'Let's face it, Boys, the only thing that's handy about Howard is that he lives round here'

I am not known for my practical skills! One day, I started painting the outside of my house in Milltown when the Boys descended on me. They would do it, they said. I asked what I should do and one said to put some Bowie on the record player and make some tea. That was when I heard the comment above.

Thanks to all the Boys and not just for painting the outside of my house! Tony is right when he said it was a privilege for me to get to know them. The Milltown Boys, with all their flaws and faults (like most of us), gave me an insight into their world that few people like me would ever be privileged to have.

I could acknowledge many people who have helped me on my journey through life – my family, the youth work community, my academic and research colleagues, the politicians and policy makers, my international friends, my fellow musicians, bikers, horse riders and footballers – but actually those I really want to thank deeply and with all my heart are the Boys themselves. As the Grateful Dead once sang, 'what a long, strange trip it's been', though they were probably referring to something else!

Howard Williamson
Treforest, South Wales
October 2020

INTRODUCTION

For 30 years, I wrote a column in a youth work magazine. One of them was about 'strange fascinations', a phrase from 'Changes' by David Bowie. It was about the intriguing observations made by young people when they were outside their familiar environments. One example I gave was the city girl in the minibus, on a youth club trip, who had never seen cats' eyes: out of the blue, as we were driving at night towards a remote cottage in Snowdonia, she observed that "they must be rich in Wales because they can afford to put lights in the middle of the road" (see Williamson 2004b).

I mention this only to make the point, right at the start, that my own 'strange fascination' with the 'Milltown Boys' may have inadvertently produced some distorted, even 'fantastic', perspectives on and from their lives, though of course I hope that this is not the case. On the contrary, I hope that my proximity to their lives and profound familiarity with their environment, over many years, has enabled me to convey a faithful description of their life course and a plausible interpretation of their circumstances, one that may make sense both to the reader who is unfamiliar with their 'life world' and to the Boys themselves. The late Peter Lauritzen, a good friend and a senior official in the youth section of the Council of Europe, to whom I dedicated my inaugural professorial lecture (Williamson 2012), complimented *The Milltown Boys Revisited* as follows:

> [it] is not only standard setting in its methodology but also an example of how *distant intimacy* like this is required in participant observation – thus it is sociology and education at the same time. Williamson does not guess about young people, he knows. (emphasis added)

I very much liked the notion of 'distant intimacy'. I hope that is what I have maintained in the production of this study, conveying the complexities and uncertainties of the life course through revealing the many interlocking and over-lapping layers that affect it.

More closely related to the Milltown Boys is a story about the BBC. Shortly after writing my first book about them (*Five Years*, published by the National Youth Bureau in 1981 and described some years later in the magazine *Young People Now* as a 'classic text'), two young BBC journalists decided to make a half-hour documentary focusing on the lives of the five 'Boys' profiled in the book: Danny, Marty, Jerry, Ted and Pete. They came to Milltown, took us to the pub and then interviewed those five individuals in a local hotel. I was paid £120 for assisting with the Radio 4 programme. It was, like all other remuneration I have ever had from the study (from writing, speaking or interviews), shared equally between us, in this case £20 each (more than a week's wages for them, at the time, though all of them were technically unemployed).

Janet Cohen (the presenter of 'Five Years' in May 1982) went on to be a regular presenter on Radio 4's *The World Tonight*. More than 25 years later, I got in touch to say that I had written another book about the 'Boys' (at the age of 40) and perhaps she might be interested in doing a follow-up programme. I had dinner with her in London and her, in principle, interest in making another programme was contingent on all five of the 'original' Boys taking part. I asked each of them. Four agreed. Jerry, as he had always been, was reticent, not wishing to expose his family to the spotlight. He declined. And so, for the time being at least, the idea was put on hold.

Then Marty, who had once asked me to lend him a 'tenner' and set the ball rolling for my relationship with the Boys (see *The Milltown Boys Revisited*, p.3), died. That was certainly the end of Janet's tentative plan.[1] However, a year after Marty's passing, I discovered that Gwyneth Williams (the producer of 'Five Years' in 1982) had become the Controller of BBC Radio 4. I sent her an email in July 2015 telling her a bit about the Boys. She wrote back, having plucked her copy of *Five Years* from her bookshelves and re-read it:

> Dear Howard – what a lovely e mail to receive … Of course I remember *Five Years* – I still have my copy of the book which I immediately got down from the shelf and looked through. What has happened to all those years …????>>>> They were such an interesting group = each full of character and so young with everything ahead of them. How kind of you to tell me what has happened to them.

1 After writing this book, I wrote to Janet to give her a short update on the five 'Boys'. This was her reply (4.9.20):

> Howard, how great to hear from you! It's lovely to know that Milltown Boys at 60 is finished but sad to hear of their problems. They seem to have had their share of troubles. It's brilliant that some of them still feel able to talk to you. I wonder what they think of the books? … Best wishes, and thanks for the update. Janet.

The following day she sent a supplementary message: 'I must sit down and read about those boys again. They were so interesting'.

In the end, the closest I got to talking, once again, about *Five Years* on the radio was when I was invited to appear on Radio 4 on Laurie Taylor's *Thinking Allowed* (3 November 2004), to discuss *The Milltown Boys Revisited*. Laurie described *Five Years* as a 'ground-breaking' study of youth and crime and seemed quite fascinated that I had managed to get in touch with them again. As the blurb for the programme reported:

> **Laurie Taylor** speaks to Dr **Howard Williamson** about his new study *The Milltown Boys Revisited*. The book is a sequel to *Five Years*, a ground-breaking study in the 1970s of a group of boys on one of Europe's largest council estates. At its close, the boys he interviewed were left with few prospects and bleak futures. In *The Milltown Boys Revisited* Williamson returns to find out what has become of them.

Ethnography is invariably a combination of two forms of data collection – participant observation and in-depth interviewing. It is considered to be an approach to research that provides a level of understanding that cannot be achieved through the use of quantitative, statistically based investigations or less immersive qualitative methods.

As an undergraduate, I took a module on 'human socialisation' delivered by the late Geoff Pearson. Geoff introduced me to 'Cultural Studies 7/8' that was, in effect, the precursor to *Resistance through Rituals* (Hall and Jefferson 1976), a collection of papers on post-War British youth culture by researchers at the Centre for Contemporary Cultural Studies in Birmingham; it was one of the main catalysts for my interest in youth studies. I also wrote an essay for Geoff on post-war British youth culture, comparing Mod and Skinhead culture through the music and art work of The Who and Slade, and the cover notes on their albums, *Quadrophenia* and *Sladest*, respectively. Geoff became a lifelong friend and I dedicated *The Milltown Boys Revisited* to him (and to my PhD supervisor, the late Geoff Mungham who, with Pearson, had edited another influential text: *Working-Class Youth Culture*). Geoff Pearson's take on ethnography, that it can never quite 'tell it like it is' (as some would claim), is precisely because the ethnographer can never see things completely 'from the inside'. Instead, through vivid and detailed descriptions, the ethnographer seeks to achieve a tension and a balance between proximity and distance, which is what I hope I have sustained through my work on the Milltown Boys:

> What is required of a good ethnographer is neither full membership nor competence, but the ability to give voice to that experience, and to bridge the experiences of actors and audiences.
>
> *(Pearson, 1993, p.xviii)*

My participant observation of the Boys in the mid-1970s focused on a group of 12 of them, including the 5, named above, who were profiled in both the book and the radio programme called 'Five Years'. The 'core five' are amongst the 'key

TABLE I.1 The Milltown Boys who were interviewed in 2000

Colin		
Ryan	*Gary*, Shaun, *Tony*, Nick, Denny	*Spaceman*
Trevor		Nathan
Alex		*Jamie*
Tommy	***Danny***	Gordon
Mark	**[Marty]**	Eddie
Matt	**Ted**	*Kelvin*
Nutter	**Jerry**	
Mack	**Pete**	
Richard		
Paul		
Derek		
Mal		
Vic		

Note: those interviewed in 2020 in italics

12' individuals who are thanked first, and separately, in my PhD thesis. Forty-one other Boys were also name-checked and acknowledged in the thesis. When I was drawing up a list of prospective respondents for my follow-up in year 2000, and consulting with Danny, he mentioned 14 more of the Boys, whom I recalled but had not known very well. That produced 67 names and the decision and determination, having learned that 7 were already dead, to try to interview half of them. My priority had been to find those I had been closest to in the 1970s but I recognised that I might need to 'top up' my respondents with some with whom I had been less familiar. Ten of the 12 Milltown Boys who were at the heart of my 1970s research were interviewed in 2000, along with 14 who I also knew pretty well. Only six were missing from my PhD Acknowledgements page in 1981, though I had known them at the time – some of them rather well (and I was surprised to discover I had overlooked thanking them). The Boys in these respective groups are listed in Table I.1, highlighting that those interviewed in 2020 are drawn, reasonably evenly, from all four groups.

In 2020, my thoughts came to focus on trying to interview about one-third of the 30 I had interviewed for *The Milltown Boys Revisited*, not so much explicitly from all four of the groups discussed above but rather from across the 'classification' I had speculated on in 2000: the 'successful' group on one side, those who have got by on the margins on the other side, and those somewhere in the middle. The caveat is that I have always argued that it is very difficult to sustain the plausibility of such classifications when one probes more deeply into individual circumstances: presumed 'success' may be tempered by experiences of relationship breakdown and mental ill-health (as in Shaun's case) or presumed 'failure' through, for example, long-term unemployment and bouts of imprisonment may be counteracted by evidence of stability in personal relationships, domestic comfort and deeply expressed personal happiness (as in Danny's case).

I first probed some of the issues I was interested in with one of the Boys who had not hitherto featured specifically in my earlier accounts, and I do not include his story in any detail here; having had a long and interesting conversation with him in the bar at one of the gatherings of the Boys, I recalled his capacity for reflection and analysis, and asked him if I could 'consult' him on my thoughts about following up the Boys and the kinds of questions I might ask them. After this, I succeeded in completing a *research interview*, lasting between one and two hours, with 12 of the Boys (for whom pen portraits are provided below). Pete asked to answer my questions by email but ultimately did not do so. However, over the years, I had also had intermittent contact with many more of the Boys, though that did not always convert into a full research interview; in contrast, in the case of two of the Boys with whom I conducted a research interview, I had had no contact whatsoever since I last interviewed them in 2000! This book is based on my uneven relationships with all of them and on information provided by them in the following ways (see Table I.2):

TABLE I.2 Contact with the Milltown Boys since 2000 and sources of information for the current book

	Contact since 2000	*Source of information*
Ted	Regular	Conversation & **Research Interview**
Danny	Regular	Conversation & **Research Interview**
Spaceman	Regular	Conversation & **Research Interview**
Marty	Regular until his death	Family communication
Gary	Regular	Conversation & **Research Interview**
Matt	Twice	Facebook & **Research Interview**
Paul	None	**Research Interview**
Richard	None	Hearsay
Denny	Rare	Hearsay
Ryan	Rare	Conversation
Tony	Occasional	Conversation & **Research Interview**
Alex	Rare	Conversation & hearsay
Mack	Rare	Facebook & **Research Interview**
Mark	None	**Research Interview**
Jerry	Occasional	Conversation
Nathan	Rare	Conversation
Shaun	None	Hearsay
Derek	Once	Conversation
Colin	None	Hearsay
Jamie	Occasional	Conversation & **Research Interview**
Gordon	Occasional	Conversation
Eddie	None	Hearsay
Nick	None	Hearsay

(continued)

TABLE I.2 Cont.

	Contact since 2000	Source of information
Kelvin	Occasional	Conversation & **Research Interview**
Trevor	Rare	Conversation
Tommy	Rare	Conversation
Mal	None	Hearsay
Pete	Once	Conversation
Vic	Occasional	Facebook, text & **Research Interview**
Nutter	None	Hearsay

Pen portraits of the Boys in this book

Ted lost both of his parents when he was a child. He and his younger sister were looked after for a while by their eldest sister (who was still a teenager at the time), but Ted's wayward behaviour led to him being taken into care. After being moved between a succession of children's homes and always being in trouble, he was sent to a 'CHE' (a community home with education on the premises). At 17, he fathered his first child, who was born while he was in Borstal and shortly afterwards he received a lengthy prison sentence. Ted's offences ranged from theft and robbery, to assault and wounding. After his spells in custody he never returned to Milltown and lives about an hour's drive away on an estate with an equally hard reputation. Ted has ducked and dived throughout his life, often but by no means exclusively in connection with the drugs culture. He has had a number of spells in prison and multiple relationships. He has 7 children and 15 grandchildren. At the time of writing the book, he was having treatment for a diagnosis of incurable but treatable cancer. He deteriorated dramatically at the start of 2021 and, alerted by some of the other Boys, I went to see him on 21 January. His last words to me were 'Take it easy, Prof'. He died the following day.

Danny spent much of his childhood living with his grandparents in Milltown. His parents lived on an adjacent council estate. In his early teens, Danny was taken into care and sent to an approved school. Initially, most of his offending relating to motor vehicle theft (cars and motorbikes) though it expanded to other forms of theft, robbery and sometimes violence. Danny progressed steadily through the custodial system – Detention Centre, Borstal and then prison. He married in between custodial sentences, then divorced, before establishing a long-term relationship with his current partner. His older daughter was born while he was in prison. He has spent most of his adult life on the wrong side of the law. In his 20s he served some serious prison sentences, lasting some years, but for some time his lower level offending has not produced any spells in custody. He still lives in the heart of Milltown, with his partner and his second child, who is still a teenager.

Gary attended the comprehensive school and was reputed to be the hardest kid from his particular feeder junior school. He was, and still is, an ardent 'City' fan and, as a teenager, was always on the fringes of a mosaic of offending behaviour, from the streets, in scruffy clothes, if he had ever been seen out at all. But here he was, dressed, as he had been before his mental illness set in, immaculately. I had prepared a slide show of old photos from the 1970s, of the Boys and their haunts, projected on to a large screen, and instructed the DJ to play music only from that era. Marty sat down opposite the screen and immersed himself in his memories of those days, as he listened to Roxy Music, Eddie and the Hot Rods, Slade and David Bowie.

I concluded my 'speech' in the church with messages of condolence from Jerry who was returning from holiday in Cyprus only that day, and from my former wife Pip, who had written some sections of *Five Years* with me (notably the chapter about Pete), knew of Marty's passing, was very fond of him, and had sent her expressions of sadness.

I had a special attachment to Marty. I saw more of him and probably knew him better than any of the other boys. I stayed in contact with him, quite frequently, well into his later years. I went to see him more than once during the spells he spent in the local psychiatric hospital. I even drove from Birmingham to visit him in Bedford prison, long after I had any 'need' to do so. Perhaps it was because he was the first of the Boys I ever met; perhaps it was because he was the first of the Boys I ever went to see in custody. Even when he was well into his 30s, I visited him in his ground-floor flat from time to time, never losing touch, and remember being deeply saddened when I was in the flat one day, surrounded by empty lager cans and empty cans of dog food (his dog had become almost his only companion), when a group of local schoolkids started throwing small stones at the windows, taunting the 'old nutter' who lived there.

After my carefully chosen words that celebrated Marty's positive character and downplayed all the other more negative things I could have mentioned (but rightly did not do so) I saw that Sandra was almost smiling amidst her tears. There was a muted and then steadily increasing sound of hands clapping, as many people applauded (Sandra thanked me later for bringing some humour and laughter into the pathos and sadness of the day). I sat down and the service continued with prayers, one more hymn and then departure from the church to Simple Minds' *Don't You Forget about Me*.

Outside the church, a woman approached me and said she had appreciated my words. I did not know her, but she told me she was Buster's sister. Buster was a contemporary of the Boys. I might easily have included him in my follow-up study; he was on the 'list' I drew up in 1999 and I had known him well in the 1970s. He was one of the key '12' (see above). Buster died of alcoholism in 2005. Others, both known and not known to me, also complimented me on my words for Marty. I felt moved and humbled. This was not my world and never had been, but clearly its people generally seemed to accept and value my presence, and indeed my contribution to their lives, even in death.

Most people at the funeral then headed straight for the working men's club in Milltown where the wake was to be held. I tracked down Jeanette and Catherine, who suggested that we went to the Crematorium. In the car we talked about Marty, of course, and about the culture of Milltown that suppressed difference, distinction and achievement. I told them about Marty, in his early 20s, embarking on a computer course at an adult education college, as part of his plan to turn his life around. I took him there on his first day and watched him walking in enthusiastically, dressed as he imagined a student should dress. Three weeks later he had dropped out, in his words because he was "stifled by my own past". He simply did not 'fit'. On the journey to the Crematorium we were sad, but we laughed too, remembering all kinds of funny moments all those years ago.

On arrival at the Crematorium, I handed over Ted's wreath [later he asked whether I had pretended it had been from me!]. The service was very short. *Calon Lan*, a moving Welsh folk tune, was playing as we entered. We placed a flower on the coffin. The vicar said a few more words in prayer. And then *Heroes* played for Marty one final time.

I hugged Sandra just after coming out. Another relative, someone I had never seen before, came up and shook my hand, in appreciation of my words in the church. A few others, also unknown to me, expressed similar sentiments: 'You don't know me, but just wanted to say…'. Then we drove back to Milltown.

The wake was something of a reunion, and I chatted with so many people. Some had already drunk too much! People I thought I did not know seemed to know me. I took a few photographs, trying not to be too intrusive. I had photocopied a collage of some poor quality but highly evocative, and now sentimental, pictures that included Marty, and I handed these to anyone who requested them. I talked at length with Gary about the working-class work ethic (Gary epitomises it), and then to Laura (Ryan's wife) about her three acres of land and the horses that they had acquired since I saw them last. I have always been made to feel so welcome. Milltown may not be my background, but there is an unquestionable affinity with many of the Boys, for whom I have the greatest affection and respect.

Inevitably, there was a lot of reminiscing, some rather superficial and sarcastic, some very poignant and reflective. Ted said that I should have been writing it all down for another book! I retorted that there was a time and place for that kind of exercise and it was certainly "not today". I was here because of my relationship with Marty, not as a researcher.

I talked to Sandra, who was getting through the afternoon magnificently and who was being watched over with care and consideration by the Boys, especially Gary, who is a gentleman personified when he so chooses, and was always close and loyal to Marty, even when things became 'too much' for most. I met friends of Sandra and discovered links and connections, through both people and the university. We talked about Clem and Nelson Mandela. Six degrees of separation is sometimes too much!

Eventually I decided to leave. Sandra was heading for one of Milltown's pubs to have something to eat and she asked me to come, but I declined. Daniel came over to say thanks for what I had said. Marty's godmother, whom I did not know, also thanked me for my words as I was heading out of the door. Ted was very, very drunk and I was convinced it was time to take him home. He was glad to have come: he and Marty were blood brothers at one time, at least for a while. I dropped him off at the pub near his house; he was still determined to have another drink!

Spaceman had left early, taking advantage of a lift from Phil. He sent me a text:

> Sorry I had to dash H. That was a great tribute to Marty of which I am sure he would have been proud. You'll have to do mine when I peg out. Take care, H. Spaceman

Ted also sent me a text the following day: 'Thanks for yesterday prof'. "We may have been little bastards, but we were little bastards with manners" was how Ryan had described the Boys in *The Milltown Boys Revisited* (p.212). In some ways, that just about sums them up.

I never really planned to write an account of Marty's funeral, but I woke up the following morning and felt compelled to try to capture the events of the previous day. It took me three hours to write. A lot of the 'Boys' in my two books about them, as well as many others, were there – in the order they are listed in *The Milltown Boys Revisited*: Ted, Danny, Spaceman, Gary, Ryan, Alex, Mack, Nathan, Derek, Jamie, Gordon, Kelvin, Trevor, Vic, Nutter – exactly half of the Boys I had written about over a decade before.

There were also some who were conspicuous by their absence. As noted above, Jerry was on holiday abroad and we had failed to track down Pete. Surprisingly, Mark didn't come. Matt, Paul, Richard, Denny, Mal, Tony (understandable, given the distance), Shaun (who probably didn't know), Nick, Tommy, Colin and Eddie were not there either.

Though Marty's funeral was not a day to be taking notes for another book, his death was certainly a trigger for thinking about it. Since 2014 I have thought about it, on and off, and consulted with the Boys about it. It was, sadly, another funeral – that of Gary's 24-year-old son, Adrian, who took his own life – that convinced many of the Boys, including Gary, that it should be done.

2

GETTING STARTED (AGAIN)

A lifetime with the Boys

> What I love about you Boys is that whenever there is something to celebrate, you all turn up; and whenever there is something to commiserate, you all turn up. I don't think I have witnessed such *loyalty* amongst friends in any other part of my life.
>
> *(Spaceman recalling my words at a 60ᵗʰ birthday party)*

I've been linked to and writing about the 'Milltown Boys' for almost 50 years. It should therefore be no surprise that various strange and interesting moments and surprises have arisen over that time. I have a colour photo of Gary, as a teenager (in 1979), looking at the pictures in my copy of *Folk Devils and Moral Panics* (Cohen 1972), about the Mods and Rockers in the 1960s. By the late 1970s, many of the Boys were second-generation Mods, attired in Parka jackets, and worshipping The Jam and The Who. Thirty years later, at a 'thank you' party I held for the Boys in 2008, following the publication of *The Milltown Boys Revisited*, Gary helped himself to a photocopied A4 black and white version of the same photograph. Gary's daughter, Simone, had apparently been very curious about that picture; at the time Gary took it home, she was doing 'A' level Sociology and knew of Cohen's study. She was all the more bemused when her teacher suggested she should read my book about the Boys!

In the early months of the year 2020, as most of the Boys were reaching the age of 60, there were two further, rather odd but fascinating experiences. In my third-year undergraduate university module on Social Policy and Young People, which I have been teaching for well over 20 years, I ask students to research and discuss the changing nature of youth transitions over three generations of their families. Ideally, male students discuss what life was like for them between the ages of around 15 to 25 with fathers and grandfathers (or equivalent), female students with mothers and grandmothers (or equivalent). Crudely speaking, for the cohort of students in question, we are talking here of a generation born around 1960, another around 1980, and a third around 2000. As evidence of their preparation, the students are required to provide me with a short profile of each of the people they have talked to. As I read the profile of someone from the oldest generation (of women), I realised that the person in question was very conceivably one of the girls who had hung around with the Boys. And, when I asked the student to delve further, sure enough it was! I was completely phased by this discovery: after a somewhat sad and certainly very wayward childhood, early single parenthood and other things that might typically have been predicted, I learned from my student that she married, went to college, trained as a secretary and spent the next 25 years in regular administrative employment. Like some of the Boys, she created a personal and occupational pathway that produced a celebration of her resilience and success, rather than an anticipated commiseration with exclusion and failure.

Ted was diagnosed with incurable but treatable cancer at the end of 2019. He found it hard to describe and discuss it in any detail; his daughter, Hayley, showed me the letter from the hospital. Danny and I went to see Ted in January 2020 and, in his house when we arrived, there was a younger man, around the age of 40. I thought it just might be Ted's eldest son, born while Ted was serving a custodial sentence in Borstal at the age of 17. I changed my mind, however, when he expressed curiosity as to how the three of us knew each other – "had we been to school together?", he asked! Before Danny or Ted could respond, I said Danny had been to an approved school, Ted to something called a community home with education on the premises and, before I could continue, Ted interjected and said I had been at a "school for fucking toffs". The four of us then went off to a local café and, as Ted and Danny were buying a second round of cups of coffee (with a drop of cannabidiol – CBD – oil for Ted), the younger man asked how long I had known his dad. It *was* Ted's eldest son after all, though clearly he didn't know anything about me (Ted normally introduced me to the incessant stream of visitors to his house as "the one who writes the books"). Apparently, Andy's mother had not revealed the identity of his father until he was 16, at which point he had got in touch with Ted. Andy himself has six children, by three different women, uncannily in that way at least following in the footsteps of his own father. When I told Andy of my connection to his father and that I worked at a university, he asked if I knew anything about criminology. His daughter, he told me, was starting a criminology degree later in the year and Andy wondered if I might be able to give her some advice!

Whether or not I am a criminologist (even if I may have studied young offenders, worked with young offenders, and chaired the Youth Crime Prevention and Inclusion Committee for England and Wales, when I was a Board member of the Youth Justice Board between 2001 and 2008) has, at times, been a matter of some dispute.[5] I have never worked in a criminology department of a university.

---

5 There is a slight edge to that remark. Just a few years ago, I was removed from a doctoral studies supervision team, at the request of the PhD student, on the grounds that I was not a 'real criminologist',

In 2020, however, as I was embarking on this study, James Treadwell published *Criminological Ethnography: An Introduction* (Treadwell 2020). It is peppered with the classic texts that I studied as an undergraduate (on modules more concerned with the sociology of deviance than with criminology, which hardly existed as a subject at the time) and which had inspired me to engage with the Milltown Boys in the first place. At the time, I had no idea that the study of the Boys would last this long. But I am name-checked by Treadwell precisely because of the longevity of my interest in and coverage of the Boys. Towards the end of his book, in a section entitled 'Longitudinal Ethnography and Time in the Field', Treadwell notes that most ethnography is relatively limited in terms of time in the field and he considers the merits of more long-term engagement, such as my own, noting that I returned to the study of the Boys 25 years after the first study, presenting

> a staggeringly diverse range of lives, and as a longitudinal picture of those involved in drug use, crime and poverty growing up (and in some cases moving on) it is fascinating and yet it gets little traction in debates about crime, rehabilitation and desistance.
>
> (*Treadwell 2020, p.176*)

Treadwell goes on to make the seductive observation that Wilson's (2007) equally unusual longitudinal ethnography, of the Northern Soul music scene, "blurs the lines between ethnography, history and autobiography in interesting ways" (Treadwell 2020, p.176).

Much the same, I would hope, could be said about the study of the Milltown Boys. As I approach the 50th anniversary of the start of the study, I am also celebrating half a century of a close relationship – a kind of friendship – with the Boys, with some obviously rather more than others. I was the best man at Danny's wedding[6] and took the photographs for Ted,[7] Jerry and Shaun at their weddings.

---

despite my range of engagement with the youth justice system, though both my colleagues in criminology and I think that the reasons were rather more complex than that!

6 I have always been particularly close to Danny, despite our completely different backgrounds, and our lives have intertwined in various ways. I once found myself brushing down his daughter Cathy's horse with him at a local riding stables. We always stayed in contact, one way and another. The strange connections that accompanied this relationship continued through to the next generation. At the age of 16, Danny's younger daughter, Octavia, was the girlfriend of a boy from my own younger children's school, whose parents were medical professionals. I always wondered how Danny presented himself to them, when they met, a topic I broached nervously with him during the research interview.

7 In March 2020, I had a message through Messenger from Ted's second child, Natasha, who I have never met: *Hiya Howard hope your keeping well, I'm looking for the books that dad is in I know one is called Milltown boys revisited but can't remember the other one I'm trying to order them see lol xx.* I wrote back saying that I had actually taken the photos at her parents' wedding. Natasha asked me if I had any of those pictures 'as my mother cut them up'. Sadly, I do not. But I did send her a copy of four of the Boys made up in Bowie's *Aladdin Sane* make-up, which she loved.

   In April 2020, I had a completely unexpected Facebook friend request from Vanessa, Tommy and Suzanne's youngest child, 20 years since I last set eyes on her. I'd talked to her when she was 14, in the garden, about the 'cultural tensions' of living in Milltown and going to an elite private school

Denny came on holiday with me, to a cottage in north Wales where we linked up with a group of student mates of mine at the end of the academic year; I'd bumped into him the day before, the start of his fortnight's holiday when he said he had 'nothing to do'. I suggested, quite spontaneously, that he came along. He got on fine with my mates and, indeed, they still ask after him.

I threw a memorable wild party in Milltown to mark my leaving the estate (Danny's parents turned up with a bottle of Laphroaig whisky for me, to wish me well, expressing the hope that I would not lose contact with their son; I never did). Later, I helped Denny's young adult son prepare his best man's speech for Denny's third wedding, spoke at Marty's funeral at the request of his mother (see above), occasionally socialised with them in a variety of other ways, and certainly went to many of their birthday and anniversary parties.

When I moved away from Milltown, some of the Boys visited me occasionally, individually or in groups; Danny and his girlfriend lived in my house for a month when I went to America in 1980. From time to time, some of the Boys have dropped by to see me ever since. Marty was one of the more regular visitors when I lived in Birmingham (until the mid-1990s). Long after the publication of *The Milltown Boys Revisited*, in 2015, Pete and his boyfriend Barry turned up one day quite unexpectedly at my house in Treforest, though at the time they were living in the Canary Islands. Conversely, when the opportunity has arisen, I have always visited some of the Boys, turning up out of the blue, or at least talked on the phone. I visited Matt in prison when he was well into his 40s and he subsequently wrote me a touching letter of thanks, for 'bothering'; in 2019, I went to see him after discovering he had had a life-saving operation. Tony and I had a lengthy mobile phone conversation after he left a message, after 16 years of no contact, on my phone, to the effect of: 'if you're not dead and this is still your number, call me back!'. I invited Spaceman to the David Bowie exhibition at the Victoria and Albert Museum in London in 2013, for which I had free tickets. I provide more detail below about some of these casual encounters over the years.

Notably, as already mentioned, I held a party for the Boys in 2008, to thank them for their trust in me. Nearly all of those I had interviewed for *The Milltown Boys Revisited* came, and many more; I plastered the wall with black and white A4 photocopies of grainy and often blurred, but immensely and intensely evocative colour photographs of the Boys that I had taken with a Kodak 110 camera in the 1970s. The best of these were also composed as a slideshow projected on to a large screen. The DJ played music only from that era. It was my contribution to an evening

---

(as Danny's older daughter, Cathy, had also done), which Vanessa was struggling with at the time and which her parents discussed at length with me during my research interview: I was talking to Tommy but Suzanne was doing the ironing in the same room and joined in the conversation – see the dialogue in *The Milltown Boys Revisited* pp.146–148. Though it was not so pronounced, I had had similar challenges, having been an 'ordinary' clever kid from a small village attending an elite direct grant school as a 'scholarship boy'. Vanessa was a 'scholarship girl'. She had appreciated my understanding of her predicament. I accepted the 'friend' request, sending my regards to her parents. She replied with a long message including the observation that 'dad still has his book'!

of reminiscence and nostalgia, with a glam rock and punk soundtrack headlined by Bowie, Roxy Music and the Boomtown Rats but also accommodating The Stranglers, Cockney Rebel, the Sex Pistols, Sham '69, and Eddie and the Hot Rods. The catering for the party was done by Mark's wife, who was later prosecuted for social security fraud and narrowly avoided a custodial sentence; she had been claiming Disability Living Allowance while doing a range of jobs for cash in hand (see below). The joke amongst the Boys was that if I had another party, and wanted Veronica to make the sandwiches again, it would cost me more because, next time, she would have to pay tax and VAT!

By the end of the party, in the function room of a working men's club in Milltown,[8] I had shaken hands with 47 of the 60 Boys whose names I had written down just under a decade earlier, in the ambitious hope that I might possibly manage to contact and interview half of them.

That closeness did not, however, always convert or revert easily into a continuing research study. After 25 years, in 2000, most of the Boys I approached did not mind talking to me once again (indeed, all of them did so, though Jerry was reticent at first,[9] and – for this study – did not want to be interviewed: when I talked to him on the phone, he said simply, "I keep myself to myself these days"). This time around, it has probably taken some four or five years of probing and consultation before I felt that the idea might be possible and acceptable. Many of the Boys were against it when I first mooted the idea; they did not particularly want to be profiled individually, as in the previous book. They were not getting any younger; there were many things that were cause for regret or recrimination.

I had to consider not only principle but also method. I mulled over the idea of doing small group interviews and having more staccato 'conversations' with them on social media. That was the start of thinking about 'data gathering' third time around. But if there really was strong opposition from the Boys to me 'writing another book', I would not do it, not because of the challenge of increasingly robust and often rather risk-averse university ethics procedures (which I know well as chair of my own Faculty Research Ethics Committee) but 'simply' out of respect for them. There would have been little point anyway, if key people were unwilling

---

8 When I called Tony, in order to invite him, he wasn't in and one of his teenage daughters answered the phone. I explained that the party was to be held in the 'West End' (the name of the working-men's club). Hanna, then aged 13, said enthusiastically 'oh, if it's going to be in London, can we come?' That just shows how far Tony's 'family of destination' had already come, from his 'family of origin' in Milltown!

9 In 2000, Jerry had initially said he did not want to be involved in any further research; later he called me and said he would take part after all. Only years later, as we propped up a bar together, did Mark explain why Jerry had at first declined. When I left Milltown in April 1979, Jerry was in the army, on a tour of duty in either Germany or Northern Ireland. When he came home, I had gone. For many years, he had been quite bitter that I had never said goodbye. That feeling has apparently calmed, but it still lingers. It has not gone away completely. Jerry did participate in a full research interview in 2000. He did not wish to do so in 2020. But he has always been unceasingly welcoming and hospitable to me, whenever I have called round for a casual conversation. He is happy enough to tell me a lot about his life; he just does not want to do a formal interview.

to talk to me. I did, however, continue to broach the thought. The green light that converted thought to action flickered first, in tragic circumstances, at the funeral of Gary's son Adrian, where Gary himself said out loud that it must be time for another book and quite a few of the Boys concurred. The light became greener when a group of us coalesced around Ted's cancer and Ted himself asked to be interviewed again, so long as I would also help him to prepare the speech he would like somebody to make at his own funeral. After all, he said, he'd always wanted to have the last word throughout his life and he saw this, perhaps, as an opportunity to set the record (and he has quite a record) straight! He now sees himself as the patriarch of a very large, extended family rather than the hard man, feared and respected in equal measure on his local patch, which was his preferred persona in his earlier days. As I have always said about the Boys, when asked to describe the way I have approached the study and my determination to capture the many nuances of their identities, they may well often be viewed by the outside world only as delinquents, drug-takers and drop-outs but, to each other, and to those closer to them, they are fathers, friends and family men.

And, of course, they are both. Navigating and negotiating between those multiple identities, and understanding the interface and interplay between them, as I note below, lies at the very heart of the story of the life-course of the Boys. As Danny and I drove away from visiting Ted soon after his diagnosis, we discussed his persona: he had appeared very relaxed and fatalistic – "it is what it is", "nothing I can do about it" – and almost proud that he had already lived rather longer than many of his brothers and sisters (and even three of his nephews). He is certainly the proud patriarch of a huge family (7 children and 15 grandchildren, and 2 great-grandchildren on the way), all of whom visit him regularly. I pointed out to Danny that this pragmatic and fatalistic attitude was a strong characteristic of the Boys when faced with adversity of many kinds: 'you've got to get on with it' – what other option did they have? I reminded Danny of the remarks he made about doing time in prison that I recounted in *The Milltown Boys Revisited* (p.94):

> Prison is always a tough place, though the Boys found ways of making it tolerable. Their public recollections of being inside *always* gloss over the more private pain they often felt about their lack of control, and the separation from their loved ones. (Danny's marriage collapsed when he was inside; Ted, Danny and Nathan became fathers while they were in custody.). Nevertheless, they had to display rectitude when they were banged up, and sustain the stories afterwards. It was the only way, it was all they could do, for, as Danny noted poignantly, 'it was all about having a laugh. That's what stopped me from going under, messing about'.
>
> *(emphasis original)*

Danny agreed that humour and misbehaviour was often just a cover and that deeper inside, below the swagger and the bluster, beyond the toughness and fatalism, deeper emotions, pain and sadness were at play. To reveal them, however, was weakness and it suggested vulnerability, so it was better to keep it hidden. There was an inherent lack of trust in other people, apart from some very close friends, because presumed 'weaknesses' revealed might be turned back on you at any time.[10] Danny said he had written about this in a song about the 'rec Boys' (recreation ground Boys) and right there, in the car, started to sing the last verse about 'hurting deep inside'. I asked him to send me the words (to be sung to the tune of *Ziggy Stardust* by David Bowie, the Boys' lifelong musical hero):

REC-BOY

1
Rec-Boy stole a car
Up all night, cruising round Milltown,
With the 8-track full blast,
Life felt so fast
No thoughts of the past
That kid was on par
And boy did he drive that car

2
Rec-Boy burgling
Climbing through an unlocked window
Takes cash and the fags
Wearing a broad smile
Life's so grand for a while
That kid was on a par
But sometimes he went too far
Meanwhile up at the Rec Ground
The Boys start sniffing glue
Hallucinations inside their heads
When the Boys were on the glue
They had no idea what they'd do

3
Rec-Boy on remand
Broke the law a bit too often

---

10 This was the first time Danny had ever really talked about this. Yet it is a characteristic more widely shared than many might imagine. One way, paradoxically, that children keep control of their lives is *not* to talk with others about weaknesses, anxieties and difficulties, in case those they share such concerns with trivialise or over-react: see Butler and Williamson (1994). It would seem that the Milltown Boys may only now be willing to talk more deeply about their lives.

> Got sent to DC[11]
> Life now seems so hollow
> Borstal and Prison will follow
> That kid was on a par
> But sometimes he'd gone too far
> Now he's got to do his time
> And pretend that all is fine
> You can't risk losing face
> So there's things you've got to hide
> Though you're hurting deep inside

I asked Danny what 'on a par' meant and he said he'd taken the expression from golf (for a while, quite a few of the Boys spent many an afternoon on a local municipal golf course; a few, like Danny, still play occasionally): it was about levelling up with other kids who always seemed to have more than them!

The Boys certainly have a significant place in my life. When I was appointed CBE in 2002, for services to young people, Denny said that I should share the honour with them because it was through them that I had got to where I was. In some senses that is true. My own academic and policy reputation is umbilically connected, in many quarters, to my study of the Milltown Boys. Ironically, it might not have been a study: instead of leaving Milltown, one of my plans was to establish what I considered to be a 'watertight' community project with Danny and me at the helm. I wanted £25,000 over three years to pilot, with equal wages of £3,000 a year for Danny and myself, an advice, information and support 'drop-in' facility for young people. My argument was that we complemented each other in every way. I had the 'knowledge' from the books; Danny had the 'wisdom' from the street. The argument did not wash with any prospective funders: they could see my merits as a graduate and a youth worker but they saw no merits in Danny, as a 'Milltown Boy' with no qualifications and a criminal record. I was very disappointed that our plan never came to fruition. Instead, I continued with research, more widely and in relation to the Boys. It has been a unique and memorable enterprise and experience.

And I have a place in their lives: I am "the one who writes the books", which as noted above is the way I am often introduced to their friends and family members who have not met me.[12] They apologise for introducing me in that way but say that it is the only way that others will realise who I am! I could say, more cynically,

---

11 Detention Centre – the 'short, sharp, shock' custodial measure – for three or six months – that replaced the use of the birch in 1948. For a critique, see Pharoah (1963).

12 When I went to see Spaceman about possibly doing some drawings, as well as the cover for the book, we were suitably socially distanced, sitting outside. His neighbour appeared and he asked me if I knew who she was. I did not. Spaceman then told her that I was 'the one who writes the books' She had read them; she was the daughter of one of Ted's older brothers!

that it is also a way of distinguishing me from their ordinary networks of friends and contacts, perhaps putting those I am introduced to on some guard as to what they say.

Lockdown Britain and my chance to write the book

The coronavirus crisis that hit the UK in March 2020 abruptly brought all existing planning, including interviewing the Milltown Boys face to face, to a halt. Events moved incredibly fast, literally day to day. Right at the start, in the middle of March, one of Ted's daughters had posted on Facebook a request that anybody coming to see her father, who was undergoing chemotherapy, should wash their hands in the sink in the downstairs toilet before going into the living room. Vic posted a comment that his intention was to visit before the end of that week, if he could get a lift. I messaged him to offer him a lift, for which he expressed appreciation, and we agreed a day and time. The following day we aborted the plan; social distancing and the self-isolation of those with underlying health issues were no longer general advice but strict (if not yet enforced) instruction.

In Treforest, the university was planning to close its doors. Ethically, face-to-face interviews were prohibited for at least the next three months, though online communication with respondents might still be possible. Still, as I indicated to university colleagues engaged in research involving interviews, in my role as chair of the Faculty Research Ethics Committee, this would need careful and sensitive consideration: topics might now have a different effect on respondents, both because of their personal situation, anxieties and concerns about friends and relatives, and because of access to technology. By the end of the week, the university had shut until at least September.

I signed up to the Treforest Covid-19 Community Support Group, of which there were more than 200 members almost literally overnight. Having already thought about attempting some 'community organising' (after all, as one of the Milltown Boys had once said when I asked him about Milltown as a 'community' and what he might do about it: "you've been studying this stuff all your fucking life, why are you asking me?"), I scanned the list to see who I might know. I did know one or two, not many, but two names jumped out at me.

One was Marty's sister, Jenn. I sent her a private message around midnight. She replied immediately, saying she had lived locally for just over a year (about a quarter of a mile from me) and that,

> we are all really good; mum finds March really difficult but we get thru it my eldest daughter finally convinced her to take Corona virus serious … my youngest is 21 in June and her celebrations are looking doubtful … Joyce [Jenn's sister] on lock done [*sic*] in Oz the world's gone mad.

I was relieved to learn that Sandra was still alive. She was now in her late 70s; I know she is 12 years older than me. As an aside, it may be of interest to note that

Jenn, Sandra and Ruby (Marty's sister, mother and grandmother) had been one of 'three generations of women' studied by Jane Pilcher for her PhD thesis (see Pilcher 1998).

The other person on the community support group was a man I did not know, but whose Facebook profile said we had two mutual 'friends'. One was the son of my first 'director', who was in charge of the Social Research Unit at Cardiff University in the 1970s. She had been *the* individual who had asked me, after I moved to Birmingham, whether or not I had ever written about my time in Milltown and who, after she read my private and personal memoir, had encouraged me to try to get it published. That was the manuscript that, with not a huge amount of adaptation, became *Five Years*. The other mutual 'friend' was one of the Milltown Boys, Mack! I surmised, on looking more closely at the individual's profile and some of his photographs, that the connections must be through sport: rugby (my colleague's son had been a stalwart rugby player) and pool – the link with Mack was more likely to be through his son, Stuart,[13] who became one of the world's leading 8-ball pool players, with many of his most notable contests available to view on YouTube. I sent Mack a message to ask whether my speculation was accurate. It was.

And, as people rallied round, thinking of those who might be having to 'self-isolate' on their own, I called the widow of the former chairman of the city magistrates, Alun Emlyn-Jones, who had always shown so much interest in the study of the Milltown Boys. She, too, was fascinated that I was seeking to talk to them once again at the age of 60 and said that, were Alun to still be alive, he would be too.

On the very first day of complete lockdown, when the Prime Minister instructed people to remain in their homes except for four exceptional purposes (food shopping, exercise, medicines and work), I called Matt, knowing he lived on his own. In fact, he was at the house of one of his children, and two of his grandchildren were bouncing on a trampoline behind him. Matt appreciated the call. I said he sounded good and he said he was in really good shape, having had a change to medication that did not make him 'mad'. He said he would be in touch in a few weeks, for a longer chat.

After one week of lockdown, I called Spaceman to see how he was coping, living on his own and knowing that he had a range of underlying health conditions. He answered the phone, but he couldn't hear me, having gone temporarily deaf in both ears. He was hoping to see a doctor the following day. However, he was concerned about going out – "if I stay in, I ain't gonna die; if I go out, with my COPD[14] – which is like emphysema, H – I've fuckin' had it". He moved into a

---

13 When Stuart was 11, he was playing for money down the pub; I was not a bad pool player (through my youth work days!), but he beat me on the black. It was a sign of things to come.

14 Chronic obstructive pulmonary disease (COPD) is the generic name for a group of lung conditions that cause breathing difficulties. It includes emphysema, which is also how Spaceman and some of the other Boys also describe their condition.

lighter mood, saying this lockdown reminded him of the Miners' Strike when there were blackouts and Prime Minister Edward Heath declared a three-day week in order to conserve electricity (1973). He recalled being at Marty's nan's house, the first time the lights went out; apparently Ruby had announced that the lights must be back on, because, in the darkness, she had seen an ice cream van, with its lights on,[15] come around the corner! Spaceman laughed at this recollection – Ruby clearly thought the street and vehicle lights were powered from the same source!

Strangely, the same evening, I also talked to Gary, holed up in his flat in Milltown. When I called, he took time answering his phone, saying he had been having "an old man's snooze". He was surprisingly upbeat about his isolation, having always been a phenomenally active and hard-working individual. He said with pride that he and his 'boys' (his workforce, who he said made great play of the fact that Gary was the old man of the team) had just finished their work on the Shard, in London, when the lockdown was announced. Yes, Gary said, it was hard to think of himself and the rest of the Boys as 'old'; in fact, were it not for the lockdown, a whole crowd of them would have been heading to Spain the following weekend (early April 2020) for Phil's stag do – he had split up with his wife and was getting married again.

Facebook links but writing doubts

Ted's Facebook page profiled his occupation as 'landing cleaner', with the equipment required listed as mop, bucket and sweeping brush. It says that he studied at 'cambrige and oxford'.

When I first read this, I sent Ted a text message saying that if he was to make these grand claims about himself he should at least spell Cambridge correctly. His reply by text was that these were prisons, not universities! And, for those in the know, 'landing cleaner' is one of the plum jobs for convicted prisoners. It is a trusted 'occupation' but it is both easy and it allows mobility within a wing, enabling messages, and sometimes contraband, to be passed. It is, arguably (if you stretch the argument far enough), commensurate with the privileges and opportunities that might accrue, on the outside, from an Oxbridge education!

I was well aware that Ted had been referring to prisons; it was very typical of the Boys to have these parodies of themselves. Another, Paul, proclaimed, under the educational line on Facebook, that he had studied how to survive life on the streets of Milltown. Mack said he worked at being unemployed!

My reticence about writing about the Boys derived not only from their own possible reluctance to take part but also because I did not want to consign them to a

---

15 They were always referred to as 'ice cream vans' and they had the same kind of musical jingle alert that they were in the neighbourhood, but in fact they were a mobile general store, selling everything from bread to confectionary to cigarettes, and sometimes more contraband produce, too.

goldfish bowl. I was acutely conscious that another inquiry into all corners of their lives might be too intrusive, however much they might willingly provide their 'informed consent' to participation in a study (as required by research ethics). I had partially felt that to be the case when I interviewed them at the age of 40 but at least, then, they had time for the consolidation of lives that had generally turned out to be reasonably satisfactory, if not – except in one or two cases – strikingly successful. The Boys had reflected on their lives to that point in a surprisingly positive way: whatever their circumstances, they could always celebrate that they were not in a worse position. So those with health problems ruminated that at least they were not dead, those who were unemployed applauded the fact that at least they were not ill, those in menial and precarious work were pleased that they were not on the dole, and so on. There was always somebody close who was worse off than them and they looked to the future hoping that they could hold on to what they'd got.

The trouble was that, 20 years later, there was probably not so long to look forward to. More were dead, had been close to death or were struggling with some level of, often serious, mental and physical illness. Many more around them were suffering in similar ways. They probably would not want me prying into the tough times they were facing, had already faced or anticipated facing in the relatively near future.

And then, out of the blue, various things happened, almost in parallel, that drew me towards the Boys once more. I had a phone call from Danny, to inform me that he was now a grandfather and that he now spent most of his time with his young grandson, Alfie. He said that he had given up drinking and that perhaps his life was turning a corner. Perhaps I should write another book, he suggested. He also told me that, since I had seen him last, he had lost his uncle, whom I had known quite well – Graham had been a removal man in 1979 and had moved my possessions, for free, to Birmingham in his van.[16] I was in Austria when Danny called and I promised to call him back when I got home.

A couple of weeks later, I had a missed call on my phone. The voicemail said it was Tony Beech – 'five-star Tony', who I depicted in *The Milltown Boys Revisited*, alongside Gordon, as undoubtedly the most successful of the Boys. I called him back, having not spoken to him for some 15 years. He said that he had been chatting with his daughter and her 'socialist' boyfriend, with David Bowie playing in the background, and they had suddenly started talking about me. We agreed to talk later in the week. I then listened in full to the phone message he had left:

---

16 I first set eyes on Danny's uncle when he was sitting on a bar stool in the Wayfarer. He was often challenged to a fight by the Boys but remained aloof and dismissive of their provocation. He only hurt people for money, he later told me. He was a hard man and a hit man, and a ladies' man. He was charming, charismatic and good company. Many years later I met him in the street. He told me that, like me, he was working at the university! It transpired that he kept the toilets stocked with towels and toilet rolls. For someone in his 50s, he said, it was a regular job – "about the only thing I can get these days".

Hi Howard … it's Tony Beech. Hi. Just came across an old CD, a Bowie CD. And I just thought, wow! it reminds me of you … Anyway, I'm glad to hear that this is hopefully a non-defunct voice message and that you're not dead, because of course you're a lot older than us! Anyhow I hope everything's good. We still live near Chester. We've got grandchildren. Time is ravaging us all, of course; we all live in shark-invested waters. Nonetheless, we're having a good time. Anyhow, if you do get this message, call me back. It'd be good to catch up.

Three days later we talked on the phone for nearly two hours, reminiscing, reflecting, bringing things up to date, discussing the state of the world and considering going to watch a game at Anfield (Liverpool Football Club's home ground, where Tony has a corporate season ticket) at some point during the coming season. He talked briefly about his particular Milltown background and connections, pondering on the current circumstances of the likes of Gary and Gordon, though he still had occasional contact with Jamie, Kelvin and, particularly, Spaceman.[17]

The following day I made a holding call to Danny, essentially promising to go to see him before the year was out. He was driving with his grandson, but had pulled in; I said hello to Alfie. Most years, I had seen Danny at least once, usually – as with Ted and Jerry, and Marty before he died – in December to wish them season's greetings.

I then called Spaceman. He was one of just a few of the Boys I had kept in regular touch with since 1999. Indeed, he had routinely come to the university to have a discussion with my students about his background and his life – a tough call (as he said, it is only one day a year where he tries to remember his past) but one that he has always discharged magnificently, testified through student evaluations of the module that invariably pointed to his session as having been the high-spot of the year. His reflective analysis is incredibly powerful, and it puts much of the academic literature about working-class culture and shattered aspirations to shame. He is one of just two or three individuals who do guest lectures for me most years (the others are a municipal head of youth services and a now retired counter-terrorism officer in the Metropolitan Police![18]).

17 It was through my research on the Boys when they were 40 that Tony and Spaceman reconnected with each other. Though they had been extremely close friends as teenagers and young men, Tony had given up on Spaceman as the latter had sunk into alcoholism and heroin addiction. But he had asked me for contact details in 2000 and they had got together, resurrecting their old friendship. They have remained in touch ever since, talking on the phone from time to time and meeting up physically at various reunions.

18 As a thank you to Spaceman, one year, in 2013, I treated him to a visit to the David Bowie exhibition at the Victoria and Albert Museum in London, together with one of the other guest lecturers for my course, a chief inspector in the Metropolitan Police. Spaceman was, at first, horrified that he could be rubbing shoulders with a cop, and did not believe that police officers could possibly like Bowie, but within minutes of introducing them, I was the odd one out. The other two got on like a house on fire, sharing their backgrounds in the Merchant Navy (Spaceman) and the Royal Marines, respectively! [The following year, they contributed to my course *together*!] We were then joined by

I opened my conversation with Spaceman by telling him that I'd been talking to Tony the previous evening. He interrupted, saying he was in Cardiff Bay with none other than Gary and Gordon (both of whom had been explicitly mentioned to me by Tony the day before)! I talked briefly to the two of them, and we all agreed to meet for a pub lunch some three weeks' hence. Spaceman was reticent about doing a lecture later in the year, saying he really did not want to do it any more (it was too hard, he said); I just asked him to think on it and tell me nearer the time. In fact, he did another session (in 2018), just a couple of days after an operation on his shoulder and despite struggling with an oxygen deficiency deriving from his emphysema that constantly left him very tired. I picked him up from his apartment and, though nervous, he said he was looking forward to doing the lecture. He had prepared some notes. In the event, he also led two seminars, responding to questions from students. And some of the students wrote to me later the same day (after he had gone home, to have a well-deserved rest), describing his reflections and contributions as 'uplifting', claiming that he had 'ignited a passion' around supporting labelled and disadvantaged young people, and that 'a glimpse of his life experience and the stuff that he faced over all these years was priceless'. Another student wrote:

> Sorry to ramble on but please let [Spaceman] know that he made a difference today whilst attending our lecture and seminar. He made me change my perspective that all young offenders are 'asbo's',[19] which is definitely not the case.

So, within just a couple of days, after a decade and a half of very limited contact, I had had some communication with 5 of the 30 Milltown Boys I had interviewed in 2000. Later that day, I saw, on Facebook, that another of the Boys, Matt, was asking his 'friends' to 'Just stop the shit I'm not dead yet'. There were a number of messages of concern and sympathy, to which I added a question as to what had happened. Matt replied:

a young woman from Latvia who was working in London for the World Association of Girl Guides and Girl Scouts. [She is now the Chief Scout of Latvia.] The four of us walked into the V&A, with me mumbling something about 'you couldn't make it up' and 'somebody should write a book about it – the cop, the crim, the Scout and the prof'. 'We need somebody to write it', I said. And the first person I met at the reception was an old school friend: Lee Child, the multi-million selling author of 'airport fiction' (see Heather Martin's authorised biography, *The Reacher Guy*, New York: Little Brown 2020).

19 ASBOs – Anti-Social Behaviour Orders – were established through the Crime and Disorder Act 1998 to deal with anybody causing 'harassment, alarm or distress'. They came to be used prolifically in dealing with young offenders and, though they were a civil offence, their breach could lead to custody. They were largely counter-productive, either because the conditions they imposed were almost impossible to meet or because they came to be considered a 'badge of honour'. Those subjected to ASBOs came to be stereotyped as acne-riddled male 'hoodies', to the point where the latter were sometimes described as 'ASBOs' – it was not uncommon to hear, in casual conversation, the remark that, for example, 'there was this ASBO in the street'.

Had an operation on my head. was in a coma for a week. you have known me as long as anyone, I'm hard to kill and I'll keep that up for as long as possible. nuff love

Following that comment, I had a Facebook friends request from Mack and then from some of the other Boys. That then became my main form of communication with them for a while. For that reason, I then spent some time exploring the presence of the Milltown Boys on Facebook. I got in touch with Kelvin because he had featured prominently in my conversation with Tony; Kelvin had once been a photographer and, like me, had held on to some pictures of the Boys in their younger days (he now keeps them on his phone). I revisited Ted's profile (which still said he had studied at 'cambrige and oxford'!). I found Vic's profile (though it was not in his own name), with a picture of him with three grandchildren, all sticking their tongues out. Richard's profile picture is a blurred image of his muscle-bound torso – huge shoulders and arm muscles, tiny waist. I also found many Facebook pages of others associated with the Boys, of the 'avenue Boys' and of the 'rec Girls'!

The norm of reciprocity

Not all the Boys were on Facebook. As noted above, Marty had died in 2014, the first of the 'core five' (Marty, Pete, Ted, Danny and Jerry[20]) to pass away and, perhaps surprisingly, the only one of the 30 I interviewed in 2000 to have died in the past 20 years. His funeral, as noted at the start of this book, was a huge event. I had been due to speak, in Bulgaria, at a major international conference on young people who are 'NEET'[21] (not in education, employment or training) but Marty's sister had been in touch and his mother Sandra, by then aged 72, wondered whether I might be willing to 'say a few words' in the church. As I have recalled above, I did not hesitate in saying that I would. I cancelled the trip to Sofia. As always, I have tried to respond positively to requests from the Boys and those around them, whenever I have been able to.

As a student, I had learned, in a course on anthropology and the sociology of violent conflict, of the 'norm of reciprocity'. I have taken a lot from the Boys, and some of them say – with a reasonable sprinkling of humour, not malice – that I have built my successful occupational career on their backs. It is rarely malicious,

20 I have always thought of them as the 'core five', primarily because they were the Milltown Boys I knew best, but also because they had featured in the BBC Radio 4 programme 'Five Years' on 13 May 1982, which I mention at the beginning of the book.

21 I am sometimes described in international gatherings as the 'founding father of the NEETs', having been one of the team that first brought what I called 'status zer0' youth to political and policy attention (see Istance et al. 1994). I don't actually like the term 'NEET', but – in the context of Marty's death and to make an in absentia contribution to the conference in Sofia – I quickly scribbled a note about Marty called 'A Lifetime NEET'. It was used in Bulgaria and later published as 'Stories of "lifetime Neets" will often end in tragedy', Children and Young People Now 29 April–12 May 2014, p.21.

I believe, because I have also always tried to give back, whenever I have had the chance or been asked to do so. That may become evident as this story of *The Milltown Boys at 60* unfolds.

Contact with the Boys since my organised interviews with them in 2000 that led to the production and publication of *The Milltown Boys Revisited* (published by Berg 2004) has, over the past 20 years, been unpredictable and sporadic, and usually quite spontaneous.

Sometimes the contact has been initiated by them, for different reasons. And though I have endeavoured to retain some level of research distance and objectivity, this has not always been easy in some instances throughout my relationship with the Boys. Even in the methodology section of my PhD thesis, I noted the impossibility of 'just letting things happen' when you have been notified *in advance* of what individuals are planning to do and what might be the likely consequences, both for others and for them, perhaps even for me. Does anyone really want to be told in advance that someone is going to break into a house, rob a petrol station, vandalise a telephone box or violently settle a score with others? I did not want to be party to such knowledge unless it had already taken place, and I took various courses of action to prevent such things happening when I knew they were being planned. I was terrified that I would be admonished for 'going native' or interfering with the 'naturalism' of the situation, but in fact my external examiner commended my honesty about the challenges of doing 'participant observation' when invariably and inevitably the researcher gets caught up in human relationships. In my own defence, beyond the personal dimensions of my intervention, I also quoted the distinguished sociologist C. Wright Mills (1970, p.215) in order to justify my actions within the context of social science and ethnography:

> It is much better, ..., to have one account by a working student of how he [sic] is going about his work than a dozen 'codifications of procedure' by specialists who as often as not have never done much work of consequence. Only by conversations in which experienced thinkers exchange information about their actual ways of working can a useful sense of method and theory be imparted to the beginning student. I feel it useful, therefore, to report in some detail how I go about my craft. This is necessarily a personal statement, but it is written with the hope that others, especially those beginning independent work, will make it less personal by the facts of their own experience.

One of the reasons I was so worried about revealing some of that personal experience was that I felt so inept and incompetent compared to the accounts of research methods recounted in published books that were similar to the initial study of the Milltown Boys that I had conducted. One of those texts was *A Glasgow Gang Observed* (Patrick 1973), which has a wonderfully systematic illustration of how James Patrick had carried out his research. Years later, I sat on a plane with 'James Patrick' (which is not in fact his real name) and he admitted, quite frankly, that he had 'tidied up' his methodology for the purposes of publication – so that his account tallied with the approaches recommended in research methods textbooks. He had written what he should have done, not what he had actually done. These days the text is typically used to illustrate the sanitisation of research methods.

Whether or not it fitted with the recommendations of the textbooks, I have always been determined to provide an honest story of the messiness of social research. It is an emotional challenge, one that becomes more powerful, demanding and perhaps even unavoidable the closer one gets to your research respondents. A lot of my research[22] has simultaneously been an intrusion into people's lives and a considerable emotional investment on my part, where there has been, in my view, some sense of moral obligation to reciprocate, if that is requested or appears to be necessary.[23] I have written about the place of feelings in social research elsewhere (see Williamson 1996). At the time, this was rarely considered, let alone discussed, but it is an issue that now seems to command some serious academic attention:

> Emotion is not an intrusion into the research process, but a constituent element of it. So why do we so often pretend it is not there?
>
> *(Loughran and Mannay 2018, p.2)*

It has even been suggested that emotions are important in the production of knowledge and add power in understanding, analysis and interpretation (see Holland 2007). Sometimes, however, it is not just emotion but also the *actions* that flows from it, arguably compromising the research process and threatening research integrity yet necessarily retaining and sustaining the personal integrity of the researcher. At least that is how it has been in my case. The most striking illustration of this in the context of the Milltown Boys relates to Spaceman's university studies. One Thursday evening, my house phone rang, around Easter time. Spaceman was distraught. He had run out of money. He wanted to know if I knew of any charities that might provide a grant or bursary to support the completion of his final year art portfolio. He only had enough money *either* for food *or* for the portfolio. Clearly, he had to eat!

Instantly, I recalled Marty's comment in the 1970s as we came back from court in the city centre. We were standing at the bus stop after a court appearance, and he asked to borrow the bus fare. I said, quite honestly, that I only had enough for myself and that I was 'skint'. Marty had laughed, almost mockingly, and said I would never

---

22 Over the years, my 'youth research' has covered young offenders, unemployed young people, young drug-takers, school drop-outs, children and young people in the public care system, young carers, all in the context of public policy development in education and training, youth justice, substance misuse and other provision supporting the transition to adulthood.

23 Even when you are not particularly close, you are drawn to the needs and circumstances of respondents. In a study I did of children growing up in maisonettes, one mother was really struggling to understand her autistic son. My father, at the time, had a role with the National Autistic Society, so I got some user-friendly material from him and made a special journey back to given them to the mother, for which she was very grateful. Social research is, at the point of data collection, essentially about *taking*; when you are asked, or see the need, to *give*, it is hard not to.

know what it was really like to be 'skint' because I would always have someone to call on or the capacity to borrow. But when he was 'skint', he had nothing – *nothing*. That day we walked the three miles back to Milltown; my bus fare bought two cups of tea on the way home.

Spaceman said that if he could not get hold of some more money, his portfolio would have to "go by the board" and he would fail his degree. I said that I did not know of any suitable charities, though they probably did exist, and anyway there would be a procedure and he would run out of time, even if the money might eventually be available. Out of curiosity, I asked how much he needed. To my surprise, and shock, because I had expected it to be much more, he said about £80.00, perhaps £100.00 at most. Of course, I knew Spaceman's history, from my research interview with him in 2000 – how he had come through heroin addiction and returned to learning. And now he was so close, and about to blow it. I said I would lend or give him the money; I couldn't bear to see him faltering now. He shouted that he had not called to beg, uttered a few expletives at me, and slammed down the phone.

I agonised over what to do. I really had admired how Spaceman had pulled himself out of the mire. After a couple of hours of thinking, discarding many options, I hit upon a plan. I prepared well. The following morning, I put on a shirt with a breast pocket, wore steel toe-capped boots, got on my motorbike and went to the cashpoint. I withdrew £100.00 and folded the five £20 notes into my breast pocket. I rode to Spaceman's first-floor flat. I rang the bell and heard him coming down the stairs. My boot was ready. He opened the door, saw it was me, and – with a growling "What the fuck do *you* want?" – tried to slam it shut. I had wedged my foot in the door and pleaded with him to hear me out. I pulled the money out of my shirt, to which he retorted, "I told you, I don't want your fucking money". I said it was not a hand out or a loan but a down payment for the first painting he would do as a graduate; if it cost more, I would pay the balance, on completion. He asked what kind of painting I wanted. I told him to use his imagination. He took the money.

Later that year, 2002, Spaceman graduated. I went to the ceremony, with an old motorbike jacket of mine in a carrier bag and a photograph of him wearing it, in the 1970s, that I had had enlarged, framed and wrapped. He greeted me with a handshake: "from one graduate to another", he said proudly. While still wearing his mortar board on his bald head, he removed his gown and put on the jacket. As he unwrapped the photo, his fellow graduates marvelled at the way he had looked when he had been their age: a better-looking version of Sid Vicious of the Sex Pistols, with a full head of spiky hair. I wondered how much he had revealed to them about the journey he had taken since then. A couple of months later, he phoned to say my picture was ready. I went to collect it – an imagined gathering of the old men with black berets and their fists in the air. It was the way Spaceman conjectured my story of having attended and witnessed the 50th anniversary reunion of a few of the surviving Spanish Civil War International Brigaders, in Barcelona in 1988. Beyond its emotional connotations for me, it is a great painting and hangs above the piano in my living room. Spaceman is convinced that I only put it up when he is paying me a visit, but that is blatantly untrue.

When the publisher of *The Milltown Boys Revisited* inquired, in 2004, about the kind of image I wanted on the cover, I thought Spaceman, by then with his university degree in Fine Art, might be interested and willing to draw something. We conferred on the imagery we wanted (a wall with graffiti; younger and older versions of some hybrid image of one of the Boys, looking at each other; some 'punk' lettering). We argued as to whether the older man should be smoking a cigarette; I pointed out that, at the time, only one of the Boys who smoked as a teenager had later given up (Jerry). We decided the older man should be reading my first book about the Boys. Over the next few days, Spaceman duly painted the cover for the book, though with a little bit of help from me. I didn't like the way he had written the title, so we glued another piece of canvas over the top left-hand corner, and I had the idea of conveying that it was an enlarged piece of the wall, so we drew larger 'bricks' and I wrote the title words like magnified graffiti.

The original 3'×2' oil painting, now hanging in my university office, was still drying at Easter time 2004 when I took it in the boot of my car to *The Fountain* pub in Milltown to show the Boys who congregated there in the middle of the day. This was the group who were mainly unemployed and still involved in criminality (shoplifting and drug dealing), the reason they were in the pub at lunchtime. Seven or eight of the Boys were there and they strolled out to my car clutching their pints. I propped up the painting. They rather liked the imagery, though one rather amusingly asked who the 'fat bastard' was, not grasping that he represented one of *them* in middle age, portrayed in the picture recalling his teenage years through reading my original book and looking at his teenage self, wearing oxblood Doc Martin's, a drape coat and a football shirt, crowned with a Bowie hairstyle! Spaceman subsequently produced some sketches for articles about the book that appeared in the *Society* section of *The Guardian*, meeting its social policy editor Patrick Butler in the process, and earning considerably more from his drawings than I have ever done from writing the book![24] Spaceman also came to London with me when the book was launched at the House of Commons, through the sponsorship of the Rt. Hon Alun Michael M.P.[25]

24 In his sessions at the university, one of the most poignant moments is when Spaceman talks about his schooldays and his aspiration to become a cartoonist, which was invariably met with derision and dismissal by teachers and careers advisers, who told him he needed to be realistic and try instead to get a job in a print shop. How Spaceman would relish contact with those who dispensed that advice, in order to tell them where they could stick it and to inform them that he had had his drawings published in *The Guardian*. Patrick Butler is still the editor of Society Guardian, remembers 'Spaceman' vividly, and was fascinated when I told him that I had written another book about the Boys.

25 Alun Michael started his working life as a journalist and then became a youth worker. He then had a distinguished political career, first as a local councillor and then as an M.P., with a range of ministerial posts (including Minister of State at the Home Office!) before becoming Police and Crime Commissioner for South Wales, a position he was still holding in 2020, when I was following up the Milltown Boys once again.

I also stayed in close touch with Danny, but otherwise generally did not have much contact with the Boys. I linked up one evening with Tony, Jamie, Kelvin and some of the other 'catholic' Boys. Spaceman and Ted came to my inaugural professorial lecture in 2012 where I introduced them to the late Alun Emlyn-Jones,[26] by then in his late 80s, who had been the chairman of the magistrates in the city's juvenile court during the 1970s when the Boys were at the peak of their teenage offending. He certainly sentenced many of them, including, occasionally, to custody. There is a wonderful photograph of them having some fruit juice together.

Some years earlier, I'd had a surprise call from Ted, 'just' to let me know that his younger sister Jacquie had passed away at the age of 36. I asked him how he was feeling and, in true 'hard shell' style, he said he was fine, and then proceeded to declare that he was not. Would he like me to attend the funeral, I wondered? He said he would. I did. Quite a few of the Boys turned up in force. They were middle-aged, still upstanding, fit and tough looking (I felt as if I was surrounded by bodyguards or security men!), and somewhat aloof, looking strong and cool. The older men, though succumbing to age (some walking with sticks), still managed to look like extras from *The Godfather*, resting on reputations built in the past. The younger ones, in their late teens and early 20s, scurried around looking 'busy', seemingly trying to build their reputations there and then, in and around the church and in the club afterwards, doing deals (largely to do with contraband cigarettes and alcohol), planning scams and smoking ostentatiously (a point I had made about the Boys themselves in *Five Years*). All dressed in black, this was a self-assured display of three generations of people living on the wrong side of the tracks.

When I was appointed CBE, in the New Year's Honours List of 2002, I was living in Denmark. One of the first people I told was Danny. I called him because I did not want the Boys first hearing about it through the media. New Year's Day is his elder daughter's birthday. She was turning ten that day. Shortly after Danny picked up the phone, I could hear her thundering down the stairs asking who it was (and presumably thinking it was somebody ringing to say Happy Birthday to her). Danny tried to quieten her down, saying it was me and that I was calling from abroad. She asked why. Danny said it was because I had just got a CBE. Quite oblivious to what that was, Danny's daughter – only familiar with three letters that referred to desirable cars and motorbikes (almost certainly through listening to her father talking): GTi, XRi, BSA – asked "how fast does it go?"

I heard, out of the blue, from Pete, living with Barry in a villa in Tenerife. Then they came back to the UK to look for a small apartment so that Barry's children, and their children, could visit occasionally. They also wanted somewhere reasonably close to an airport, to make the journey between the UK and the Canary Islands

---

26 Alun Emlyn-Jones died in 2017 at the age of 93. He was a wonderful man and a dear friend. Having often chaired the bench when many of the Milltown Boys were being sentenced, he showed a great deal of interest in their subsequent lives, knowing full well that, as he often put it, 'there, but for the grace of God, go I'. His autobiography, about a life of privilege and service, is aptly titled *A Torn Tapestry* (Pen-yr-Enfys Press).

more manageable; Barry is more than 15 years older than Pete. Pete and Barry showed up at my house in a rather grand vintage Jaguar (up for sale, for £6,000). They took me out to lunch.

I went to see Jerry, who had retired. He told me some fascinating things about the 'work capability assessments' he had undergone in order to retire (see below). More significantly, he and his wife, Sam, recounted how dramatically and drastically public sector austerity measures since 2010 had severely reduced the quality of life of their profoundly disabled adult daughter, Rachael. She was now almost completely housebound, whereas previously some social contact and activity had been enabled by social services.

Gary, who spends much of his time working in London, linked up with Spaceman and took me out for lunch one day. I called in on Ted from time to time. I bumped into Vic by the central railway station and had an interesting conversation with him about his volunteering work with the homeless (see below). There were other brief encounters, unexpectedly, with some of the other Boys – at a city farm, on the train, at the airport and in the shopping centre. But these involved only very fleeting conversations.

There had, therefore, been *some* contact and so perhaps some basis for not reappearing 'out of the blue', should I decide to conduct yet another study of the Boys.

But had such a study been done before?

Around the time *The Milltown Boys Revisited* was published, I spotted a lecture taking place in London to promote a book called *Shared Beginnings, Divergent Lives: Delinquent Boys to age 70* (Laub and Sampson 2003). I was fascinated, jumping to the false conclusion that it might be something similar, methodologically, to my study of the Milltown Boys. I imagined some grizzled old professors who had followed a group of 'delinquent boys' through life for considerably longer than I had. One of the authors was coming to London to talk about the book, so I went to hear him speak. John Laub, it turned out, was in fact a relatively young professor from the University of Maryland who, some years before, had stumbled upon the archived files from the famous *Unraveling Juvenile Delinquency* study (Glueck and Glueck 1950), a huge comparative study of 1,000 men who had been delinquent boys in the 1920s.[27] Laub and his colleague Robert Sampson sent research assistants to track some of them down and those they found were interviewed for a relatively short time largely about their employment, relationships and military service histories. What an only partially fulfilled opportunity! While Laub and Sampson's sophisticated analysis points powerfully to the simple and rather predictable finding that desistance from crime is strongly swayed by securing and keeping *work* and having the love of a good *woman* (as well as, in the USA, having served in the

---

27 Unknown to me, Laub and Sampson had already published a re-analysis of the Gluecks' data set (see Sampson and Laub 1995).

military), the Milltown Boys' study also suggests that many other tentative and extraneous factors and experiences can influence the pathways taken by those with a history of, and perhaps a propensity to (and certainly an aptitude for) offending. I am now close to being that grizzled old professor that I had presumed John Laub was. Unlike Laub and Sampson, however, who built their important study on the original data of others, I really am writing about delinquent boys to age 60 whom I have followed *throughout* their lives and whose lives I have explored in fine and calibrated detail.

A slice of history

The Milltown Boys lived through interesting times, especially for men of their social class. They were born at a time that presaged the 'embourgeoisement' of the working class (Goldthorpe *et al.* 1969), where many workers achieved an 'affluence', not only through the proclaimed social mobility of the 1960s, but through well-paid jobs on, for example, car production lines. The parents of the Milltown Boys were, however, not generally the beneficiaries of such opportunities secured through powerful trade unionism and collective bargaining. In contrast, they had often (perhaps even 'usually') remained part of the lumpen-proletariat: social geographers, writing in the early 1970s, recorded that no more than 4% of the population of Milltown could be considered middle-class; of the remainder, 19% were skilled working-class, 46% were 'other working-classes' and 31% were at the lowest level of subsistence (Herbert and Evans 1974).

The Boys themselves, as they knelt on the floor in my living room and made their own version of a Monopoly board from an old Weetabix packet in 1976 (which was a fascinating insight for me as to how they rated different parts of the estate), substituted the waterworks and electricity company for the local paper mill and brewery. These were the two most significant employers of men from Milltown, in official employment terms at least, though the holy grail of work was the massive steelworks on the other side of the city (only Nutter, amongst the Boys, ended up working there, at least for a while). Other than that, the Boys' fathers tended to work in more casual jobs, particularly on building sites.

The 1970s were halcyon days for the Boys. Technically at secondary school, but recurrently 'mitching' (skiving) off, earning money through odd jobs and helping out but otherwise generally 'having fun' (legally and illegally), most recall the long, hot summer of 1976 as a kind of 'dreamtime', almost discarding the court appearances and occasional spells in custody from their memory. They lived for leisure, doing as they wished and seemingly without a care in the world. And yet, that world around them was changing dramatically, not least in relation to the disappearance of the unskilled youth labour market to which most of the Boys aspired and for which they were destined. Their celebration of macho, machismo and manualism (the trilogy celebrated by the 'lads' in Willis' (1978) classic text *Learning to Labour*, considering how working-class kids got working-class jobs) was not preparing themselves well for life on the factory floor or on the building site, as Willis had contended, but for a future of unemployment. But they didn't really pause to think about that. Their transitions from school to work were similar to what Ashton and Field (1976) depicted as the 'careerless' – an unplanned step from a failing and failed school experience to any job available through word of mouth, the careers office or the Job Centre. The Boys were the first generation of casualties of the post-industrial society and, as I realised later (one of the reasons I decided to 'revisit' them), the first generation of the group who came to be referred to as 'NEET' (Not in Employment, Education or Training).[28]

Even the Miners' Strike of 1984–1985, though a seminal moment in British history and an event that transformed the lives of those only a relatively short drive away from Milltown, did not resonate deeply with the Boys. By then in their mid-20s, many of the Boys had already 'gone missing', as those settling into young adulthood and parenthood were described by those who were still mainly in the pub. Both groups were largely disinterested in what was going on in the wider world. If they had any politics within them, it leaned towards the right. They were concerned about immigration and its assumed effects on job opportunities. They saw some of their parents exercise the 'right-to-buy', an option a number of the Boys themselves took up not long afterwards. Paradoxically, in some ways, many of the Boys were libertarian individualists, believing that people should just be allowed to get on with things as they wished to and as best they could. The Boys opposed regulation and instruction, whether from parents, politicians, employers or trade unions. From the early days of 'liberating' boxes of fruit from the local wholesale market (where many of them worked straight after leaving school) to later days of manipulating the social security system (see below), the Boys seized self-serving opportunities when they could and tried to keep their heads down until such moments presented themselves. Even many of the more law-abiding amongst the Boys could still not resist, if they got the chance, being 'hawks' and 'wolves' throughout their working lives (see Mars 1982): you seized the moment, because there was no one else who would help you out.

Modernisation of various kinds had the effect of cramping some of their styles, especially those living on the edge. Credit cards replaced cash, pin-codes replaced signatures, people no longer had meters for gas and electric in their houses, car radios became integral to dashboards, police helicopters strengthened surveillance, and alarms on cars and in factories were becoming more sophisticated. The Boys had to think hard about different ways of getting by, inside both the formal and

---

28 The original research study about this group (Istance et al. 1994) referred to them, technically, as 'status 0', in relation to young people in education (status 1), training (status 2) or employment (status 3). I then started to depict them as 'status zer0' – a metaphor intended to convey these young people as 'counting for nothing and going nowhere' – but a senior Home Office civil servant, John Graham, decided, in March 1996, that this term was "going down like a lead balloon" in government policy debates; he proposed replacing it with 'NEET', a designation that was cemented through a subsequent government report launched by Prime Minister Tony Blair, on which John had taken the lead (see Social Exclusion Unit 1999).

informal/illegal economies. Drugs markets became more attractive, but also more competitive and more brutal.

By the Millennium, as *The Milltown Boys Revisited* recounts, the Boys had broadly taken three paths towards middle age. Firstly, there were those who had settled down with a long-term partner, had a relatively small number of children, desisted from offending, secured reasonably stable employment, become owner occupiers, and somewhat moderated their tobacco and alcohol consumption. These individuals had seized opportunities that they could not have envisaged or imagined in their youth – well-paid and relatively secure employment, foreign holidays, houses with conservatories and professional friends. [I have stayed well connected to this group, primarily offline, though invitations to their gatherings.] On the other side were those who continued to have volatile and erratic relationships, who have fathered quite a number of children by different women, operated on the margins of the legitimate economy or remained immersed in illegal activities, still lived in council (social) housing, and carried on consuming inordinate quantities of substances, not just cigarettes and alcohol, but a cocktail of illegal drugs. These individuals were the socially excluded, though rarely the socially isolated, following in the tracks first established in their youth, characterised by delinquency, ducking and diving, and detention. [I have also stayed close to this group, both offline and online.] In the middle were a more ill-defined group, often still living with the same partners but in rather distant relationships, who have earned their living legitimately through a sequence of different kinds of employment, have not been actively involved in crime but were certainly not divorced from it, lived in social housing, and still usually drank and smoked heavily. [I have lost contact with many from this group, though I have retained some links through Facebook.]

There were, of course, many nuances and exceptions to these stereotypes. As noted in earlier writing about them before they reached the age of 40, three of the Boys had achieved university degrees, four no longer lived in or very close to Milltown (and had not for many years), and seven of them had no children.

(Twenty)-Five Years

When I published an account of the Milltown Boys in 1981, documenting their lives between 1973 and 1978 (from age 13 to 18), the purpose of that book was to suggest that from a remarkably homogeneous childhood base, the teenage years had produced some striking divergence. The focus of that first book was essentially on five of the Boys – Danny, Marty, Jerry, Ted and Pete. The one-page conclusion (*Five Years*, p.115) is probably worth citing almost in full:

> If you had met them when they were 13 or 14 years old you would not have hesitated in linking these five boys together. At the time they always went around in a group – having a laugh, hanging around and committing offences together. This particular group encompassed a series of overlapping and longstanding personal friendships: Jerry and Pete, Danny and Ted, Ted

and Marty, Danny and Jerry … and so on. Within five years they had gone very different ways.

These five boys came from within less than a mile of each other and their lives had followed a similar course until their mid-teens. Yet within two years the courses of their lives were on very diverse routes. Detention Centre had reformed Pete and opened his eyes to cruelty, injustice and oppression, but it had little effect on Danny; and while it distressed Marty while he was actually 'inside', it had very little long-term deterrent effect. Similarly, the experience of prison made Danny think very seriously about 'calming down', but it simply hardened Ted. Court appearances were traumatic for Jerry, an occupational hazard for Marty and a regular part of life for Ted.

Jerry, Danny and Pete all worked when it was necessary to do so; they were also 'honest' about their actual criminal involvement. Ted and Marty were incurable skivers and pathological liars. But these two boys pulled the girls at the earliest age and became attached to individual girls long before they were 16. Although Danny was always the focus of girls' attention, he had no time for them at that age. Pete never had a girl, while Jerry's 'success' was limited to infrequent one-night stands. Jerry and Pete are quite law-abiding today. Danny does his best to stay out of trouble, but still lives on the fringes of the criminal world. Marty will always stick to his speciality of burglary and Ted forever increases the range of his criminal convictions.

So the comparisons can go on. I have not attempted to explain why such changes occurred. What I have done my best to do is to describe the cultural context in which these boys grew up and in which this behaviour and these transitions took place; and where appropriate to explore possible reasons for their differential development, such as family influences, peer group expectations, or personal anxieties. I could never be certain that such a description even covers every possibility, but I have tried to capture the critical 'locations' which were so important to the boys.

Twenty years later, as the Boys followed their very different life-course pathways and trajectories, I tried once again to explore, and have a stab at explaining, how their lives had unfolded. And, perhaps rather foolishly, I suggested that by then it was a time of consolidation – wherever the Boys had got to, they hoped to maintain that position and not slip 'back'. They seemed relaxed, if also somewhat fatalistic, about the point they had reached in their lives. One of the paradoxes about the Boys' own accounts of their lives is that, invariably, they do not complain. Their reference points are always those individuals they know who have fared, in one way or another, worse than themselves: 'at least I'm not dead', 'at least I'm not a nutter', 'at least I'm not in prison', 'at least I've got a job'. There is always someone pretty close to them in a considerably worse predicament.[29]

29 This arguably rather 'optimistic' self-assessment of their lives is in stark contrast to the perspectives of some of most privileged young people on the planet, the first generation of 'global citizens', who

There follow some extracts from the conclusion to *The Milltown Boys Revisited* (pp.236–238):

> The Boys' worlds have been made for themselves by themselves. They have endeavoured to make the best of the situations they encountered, and generally feel they have done pretty well in the circumstances. In view of the starting points in their lives, most believe they have battled reasonably successfully against the odds. Indeed, given the prevailing social and economic circumstances they experienced as children, most *have* done reasonably well, for, whether legitimately or illegally, or on the borders, they have found ways of 'getting by'. Some, however, have succumbed to adversity, though many, quite justifiably, maintain that at least they have survived, while a few have patently done rather more than that.
>
> Caution must [therefore] be exercised in passing judgment on the Boys on the basis of some extraneous measures of success (or failure), for the most significant finding from this study is the complex interaction between the life-course trajectories in the public domain and those within more private spheres. These have knitted together in multiple ways for the Boys, both positively and negatively, shedding light on the urgent need to *relate* trajectories in, for example, the labour market to those in, for example, family life, and casting doubt on the credence of analyses which do not do so. It would be so simple to portray the lives of the Boys as delinquents, drug addicts and dropouts, invoking appropriate theories of deviance and social exclusion, but the issues and explanations underpinning such processes are integrally tied to the lives of the Boys as fathers, family men and friends. These latter roles influenced, and were influenced by, the former – sometimes propelling or sustaining the Boys' criminality, substance misuse, and economic activity on the edge, though equally, sometimes causing them to refrain and desist from such activity, and move in a different direction. Similar arguments can and should be applied to relationships between the housing and labour markets and, indeed, health behaviours and leisure. It is a complex spider's web, within which cause and effect is often difficult to ascertain, but where the interaction is absolutely evident, though invariably suppressed when attention is given solely to one 'strand' or another.
>
> *(emphasis original)*

---

speak multiple languages, possess numerous high-level qualifications, and already have and are further developing valuable social networks and connections. For the past ten years I have spent some weeks each summer at the European Forum Alpbach with those young people and in the presence of Nobel laureates, ambassadors, presidents and celebrities. The 800 students who come to Austria each year routinely bemoan the fact that they struggle to secure a foothold in the labour market that is commensurate with their talents and their efforts. *Their* reference points are invariably those 'better off' than they are, or are likely to be. I have concluded that they look 'forwards and up'; the Milltown Boys look 'backwards and down'.

I was naïve, however, to think that, somehow, the Boys' lives would simply continue in the same furrow – whichever furrow they had ploughed up to the age of 40. Another 20 years later, their life stories are full of surprises once again. The social and political context could not be more different from those early days in the 1970s when I hung around the streets and the woods with the Milltown Boys. We have all lived through the 'Third Way' (see Giddens 1998), witnessed what came to be known as 'globalisation' with free trade and cheap travel, heralded the onset of populism and fake news, taken sides on 'Brexit' as the UK left the European Union, and – in 2020 – faced the national global crises that have arisen from the coronavirus pandemic.

An oral history?

I had never anticipated carrying out a *de facto* oral history with the Milltown Boys. Yet, by a quirk of fate, I had inadvertently prepared myself for it. In 1981, two years after I had left Milltown and moved to Birmingham, I stumbled, quite by chance, on a neighbour who had fought in the Spanish Civil War. While fixing up an old Norton Dominator motorbike in a garden 'shed' (in fact a very well-equipped workshop) down the road from where I lived, with a young motorbike enthusiast who had also started working on his own BSA Starfire 650,[30] for which we had to make room, I moved a cardboard box of 'junk' and spotted a small framed image of a fist surrounded by the words 'Voluntarios Internacionales de la Libertad' (International Volunteers for Liberty). I had studied Spanish at school and knew that this had something to do with the Spanish Civil War. I turned the plaque over and it was inscribed with the words:

> The Walsall Communist Party requests the pleasure of Mr Edward Smallbone at a dinner to commemorate the 30th anniversary of the outbreak of the Spanish Civil War.

The 'old man' in the house (aged 72) confirmed that indeed he had been 'in Spain', though when I went to talk to him about it, his opening remark was "of course I had not long been back from Russia" (where he had attended the Lenin International School between 1935 and 1937, though he honoured his oath of secrecy about that and did not reveal it to me until a month before he died). Subsequently, I interviewed him about his life and, in the process, read copiously about recording history through the memories of those who had lived through it. In particular, I read the seminal texts by George Ewart Evans (1956, 1987) about Lincolnshire agricultural workers and, arguably the classic of them all, *The Voice of the Past*, by

---

30 I had become a volunteer youth worker when I moved from Milltown to Birmingham in April 1979. When I acquired the Norton Dominator 600 (though with an SS650 engine), a former youth club member – who relished restoring old British motorbikes – offered to help me do it up. We pushed it down the road to the 'shed', which was in the garden of the house belonging to his girlfriend's grandfather. That was the connection.

Paul Thompson (1978). I read a lot more besides because the man I wrote about, Ted Smallbone (see Williamson 1987), embodied a particular left-wing twentieth-century history: the General Strike, a member of the Shop Committee as Cadbury's moved from manual to mechanical production of chocolate, Soviet Russia under Stalin, the Spanish Civil War, an engineer in World War II and so in a protected trade yet recurrently sacked for being a member of the Communist Party until Hitler invaded Russia in June 1941. I spent a year tape-recording Ted's life story, once a week, 45 minutes at a time. And each week I read around the historical moment that he had been describing, whether it was about the post-World War I Dalton education system, the intellectuals who fought in Spain (Ted became close friends with David Haden Guest and was with him when he died in Spain, on Hill 481 in the decisive Battle of the Ebro; Hugh Thomas (1979, p.841) describes Haden Guest as the "inspiration of a whole generation of communists at Cambridge"), the Campaign for Nuclear Disarmament (CND) peace marches of the 1950s, or the formation of the National Pensioners' Convention by the legendary retired trade union leader Jack Jones, who had also fought in Spain. Jack Jones was in the bar in Barcelona in October 1988 when I reunited Ted, after 51 years, with American International Brigader Ed Balchowsky,[31] with whom he had walked over the Pyrenees in November 1937.

It was the story of a rather chaotic gathering of a small number of surviving former International Brigaders, to commemorate the 50th anniversary of the final march of the International Brigades (which had taken place in Las Ramblas in Barcelona in 1938), that I recounted to Spaceman many years later and which formed the basis of the painting he did for me after graduating in Fine Art in 2002 (see above).

Paul Thompson (1978, p.165) wrote that,

> There are some essential qualities which the successful interviewer must possess: an interest and respect for people as individuals, and flexibility in response to them; an ability to show understanding and sympathy for their point of view; and above all, a willingness to sit quietly and listen.

I had sat quietly and listened to the *individual* life-course stories of the Milltown Boys in 2000. By 2020 I was ready to sit quietly and listen again to their perspectives on the *collective* life-course of the Boys, as well as their own more personal reflections.

---

31 Another 'strange fascination' that loops the loop in this part of the book is that Balchowsky provides me with a link to the famous American social commentator and oral historian Studs Terkel, the author of many books, including *Hard Times*, *Working* and *Hope Dies Last*. Balchowsky had been one of the Beat Generation, friends with Jack Kerouac and Allen Ginsberg. Studs Terkel did the oration at his funeral. When Ted Smallbone died, his widow asked me to make a speech at his funeral. As thanks, she gave me his Spanish Communist Party membership card and the Roll of Honour that Labour Party leader Clement Attlee presented at Victoria Station to returning British International Brigaders in December 1938.

I was well aware, of course, that the Boys, many of whom have lived less than salubrious lives, were very likely to provide justifications and to sanitise some of their more unsavoury and unpalatable behaviour. Criminologists are well versed in discussing contemporaneous 'vocabularies of motive' and 'techniques of neutralisation'. I had asked the Boys, in *The Milltown Boys Revisited*, both to look forward and to look back, which they were generically reluctant to do. Many of the Boys have lived in a narrow window of time, avoiding a gaze on what has been a past riddled with trauma, both experienced and caused, and not wishing to look too far into the future, because it is too unpredictable, especially for those living more precarious lives on the wrong side of the law. There was never much point in planning and booking a holiday in advance; tomorrow could be the day they are arrested and remanded in custody. This time, I decided to avoid asking them to dwell too much on the past nor to contemplate the future, unless they spontaneously decided to do so, and instead to consider their recollections of their relationship with me over the years.

Trusting their stories?

A criminology colleague of mine once asked me for advice on a paper she was preparing on the honesty of the accounts of criminals about their lives. I suggested that she called the paper 'Don't let the facts get in the way of a good story', recalling that the Milltown Boys were masters at the embellished anecdote and the distorted narrative, either to position themselves more centre-stage or to keep themselves more in the shadows, depending on the purpose of the story.

There has always been some concern about the reliability of memory in recounting and accounting for the past. One might ask, does it matter? I suppose it depends on what you are seeking to achieve. Gittens (1979) makes the important distinction between memory of facts and memory of beliefs and actions: it may not really matter whether or not facts are recalled accurately, for they can be checked through other sources. It is quite another matter asking people what motivated them to behave in certain ways 20 or 40 years earlier; we certainly cannot be sure that whatever they say is actually what informed their actions immediately before or during the event in question. But it is quite reasonable, once more, to ask, does it matter? In his interviews with former members of the youth organisation the Kibbo Kift, up to 50 years since they were involved, Mark Drakeford[32] (1997, pp.26–27) writes:

> Motivation is especially vulnerable to reinterpretation as individuals respond to the need to make sense of their own histories and to do so in the context of the social changes which have gone on around them. For the purposes of this study, the interplay of individuals seeking to make 'meaningful myth' out

32 The same Mark Drakeford who later became First Minister in the Welsh Government.

of their lives (Lieberman and Tobin 1983) and processes of 'collective social memory' (Griffiths 1989) has significant advantages. What we are about is not simply a history, but also a fable. The fable arises from the way people recount their past, the choices they make in remembering and forgetting.

Drakeford goes on to draw thoughts on this matter of remembering from Andrews (1993), who studied 15 individuals who had a lifetime of commitment to progressive social change. She argues that "the way in which a life is recalled by the person who lived it is as important as what actually happened during that life" (Andrews 1993, p.63).

Though they were lives lived in very different ways and very different circumstances, all these points are especially pertinent to the current study. Indeed, the Boys have always been particularly adept at spinning a good story. Danny, when interviewed in 2000, sat on the other side of the table with a spliff. I asked him why he had to smoke it in front of me. He said he needed to concentrate and collect his thoughts in order to tell me the truth; the only other times he had been interviewed was either by the police or social security officials! In both cases, he said, he had always had to construct stories that were invariably a pack of lies. So, in the case of the Milltown Boys, Drakeford's contention about memory producing fables ('meaningful myths') is therefore especially apposite. The Boys would, for sure, confirm that you should never let the facts get in the way of a good story!

And so, long before I read Treadwell's assertion that longitudinal ethnography should be considered a mixture of autobiography, history and ethnography, I was ready for this! As the old dictum goes – 'if you want to know something about somebody, why not ask them? This may not be the last word on someone, but it certainly should be the first one' (George Kelly). The pioneering oral historian and storyteller George Ewart Evans had first suggested in relation to agriculture that you should 'ask the fellows who cut the hay', a message repeated by the historian Gareth Williams (2017) in his tribute to Evans, when he wrote that if you want to learn about mining, 'Ask the Fellows who cut the Coal'. I asked the Milltown Boys to tell me about their lives, ones that had started in the homogeneity of working-class childhoods on a deprived council estate and unfolded in myriad, often quite unexpected and certainly unpredictable, ways.

A stranger's eye

The sociological imagination is routinely described as a way of 'making the familiar strange'. I certainly was a stranger in a strange land throughout my time with the Milltown Boys and though I became very familiar with their lives in some ways, I remained inquisitive and curious simply because I never quite managed to understand what made them tick. And it seems that I also provoked *them* into reflecting more deeply on their lives: I also helped them to make the familiar strange.

After a very long research interview, Gary called me the following day:

> H, I could hardly sleep all night. I've been thinking about everything we talked about yesterday. And I've realised how much we take for granted, until you start asking questions about it. I've been thinking about all the Boys and how we've stuck together, through thick and thin. And it's great you're writing about them, H, it's great. But the thing is, H, it's not just about us. It's as much about *you*.
>
> You're part of it, H; you're part of us, H – don't forget that. You've got to put yourself in the book, because it's also about who you are. Just think about it. You came out here when you were 19. Nineteen! A fucking posh-speaking university student. You should have had your head kicked in. But you didn't. Why didn't you? Because you connected with us. You knew how to relate to us, how to get on with us. You did things for us. You did things with us. But you weren't stupid. You didn't go out robbing with Marty, or anything like that. But you did get to know our world; and we let you get to know our world. You've got to tell that bit of the story.
>
> *(notes from phone call 25.4.20)*

I felt that this was quite an accolade and was rather moved by it. And I guess it does capture something of a truth that, so often, social researchers do not write about. We don't have some magic key to the worlds of others; they have to let us in.

Furthermore, once 'let in', whether or not we want to affect the lives of those who let us in, we invariably do so. Another of the Boys, after being questioned and challenged by me for an hour and a half, said, somewhat unexpectedly, "It's been an emotional experience". I asked why. Rather as Gary had said that he took so much for granted about his life, the comment this time was that it was "a bit like the dark side of the moon" – he said that I was "shining a light on things we'd never otherwise think about".

Glenn Webbe, the first black rugby player to play for Wales and himself a boy from Milltown of the same age as 'the Boys' and a close friend of some of them, recalls in his autobiography:

> the area was deprived but it seems to me now that it was quite an education growing up with such people, getting along with one another and making do with what little we had; it made you grateful for whatever it was. Making do and taking care of what you've got. As kids you knew no different, it was always a struggle without realising you were struggling.
>
> *(Webbe 2019, p.18)*

The Boys sometimes talked about Glenn, a real golden boy from the neighbourhood alongside pop star Shakin' Stevens, radio and TV presenter Jason Mohamed and Gary Lineker's second wife, the model Danielle Bux. In his book, Glenn says that he ran back and forth to school in order to save the bus fare. The Boys recall this vividly, when discussing and describing his pace, commenting that he used to run faster than the bus. He certainly ran fast through the streets and through the gulleys,[33] just like many of the Boys as they ducked and dived on the estate. Glenn concedes that he got into some mischief during his childhood and much of that was closely associated with some of the Boys.

33 Gulleys were narrow passageways between, behind and alongside housing that provided entry to the back gardens (and coal scuttles) of terraced houses or connected neighbouring streets. Many are now blocked off or gated and padlocked (for 'community safety' reasons), but in the 1970s they were open, if often overgrown, and provided an alternative set of routes through the estate – sometimes to get to, or get away from, dubious activities.

3

METHODOLOGY

"You're part of it, H", Gary had said and, of course, I am. There is a mountain of literature on the qualitative research methodology that broadly relates to the approaches I have used in my study of the Milltown boys. This ranges from relatively brief, but perhaps still rather sanitised, notes on method in a multitude of ethnographic studies, to dedicated textbooks on highly specialised dimensions of qualitative inquiry.

As already noted, I have favoured a deeply interpersonal and reciprocal engagement with the Boys. Indeed, at a 60th birthday celebration for Spaceman, suitably socially distanced in a park shortly after the partial easing of the Covid-19 lockdown, some of the Boys asked me how the book was going and explained to others who were there that I had been 'following' them for almost 50 years. It made me feel like a stalker! Another of the Boys piped up to say that, although I wrote books about them, I was a 'friend', to which another retorted that this was 'not exactly' true but that, over time, "H has become one of us". Such ambivalence has always hovered above and around my relationship with the Boys, as I explain towards the end of this book. Here it is perhaps useful to outline briefly some academic justification for the 'distant intimacy' that I introduced right at the start.

When I first wrote about the Milltown Boys, I always pointed out how I had immersed myself in their lives. This, at the time, was subjected to considerable academic criticism – that I had 'gone native' – but such criticism has become more muted over the years, acknowledging that ethnographic inquiry cannot but connect in a human relational way with so-called research subjects, though nor can the researcher ever wholly divorce themselves from their position of the inquirer. As Connelly and Clandinin (2006, p.480) argue, "inquirers are always in an inquiry relationship with participants' lives. [They] cannot subtract themselves from the relationship". There is an inevitable interweaving of the personal and the professional that can be difficult to disentangle, though consciousness and reflexivity about this duality is critical if the relationship is to be sustained at both levels. My view is that it might be possible to shed the research relationship and continue interaction at a personal level, but the evaporation of the personal relationship would quickly lead to the closure of any possibility of sustaining a professional relationship. As I have said, and as we shall see more of, the Boys saw me as an asset, even (in one case) a 'blessing' because, in a variety of ways (including 'just' listening to them), I gave something back. Mahoney (2007, p.589) suggests that it is important not to "blur the lines between our friendship (private intimate relationship) and our research collaboration (public fieldwork relationship)". I do not think some blurring of these lines can possibly be avoided, but honesty about which side of the fence the researcher may be sitting at particular moments is essential. At Ted's sister's funeral, he did not want to think that I was there taking notes, even if he quipped with some younger relatives that they needed to be careful what they said because I was likely to write it down.

Throughout my life, both in research and other arenas, I have always been attracted by the Native American proverb that you should never judge another person until you have walked a mile in their moccasins. I was, therefore, pleased to learn that Spradley (1979, p.34) adopted similar thinking in his classic text on ethnographic interviewing:

> I want to understand the world from your point of view. I want to know what you know in the way you know it. I want to understand the meaning of your experience, to walk in your shoes, to feel things as you feel them, to explain things as you explain them. Will you become my teacher and help me understand?

The Boys were my teacher from the day I met them and have continued to be so to this day. I have *always* expressed appreciation of my dual education – both an elite privileged education at a leading direct grant school[34] and through the Boys on the streets of Milltown. The Boys often see the world very differently from me and I have gained a lot from gleaning their perspectives, reflecting upon them, trying to understand them and communicating them to those who will never have that kind of 'distant intimacy' with such a group of people over such a period of time.

---

34 Alumni in former times include the author J.R.R. Tolkien (author of *Lord of the Rings*), theatre critic Kenneth Tynan (the first person to say 'Fuck' on television), politician Enoch Powell (most famous or notorious for his 1968 'Rivers of Blood' speech), and comedian and ornithologist Bill Oddie (one of 'The Goodies'). Some of those who were contemporaries of mine include fiction writer Lee Child, the first British chess grandmaster Tony Miles, football expert Simon Inglis, politician David Willetts, BBC Director-General Tony Hall, Chairman of the Victoria and Albert Museum Paul Ruddock and the first Mayor of the West Midlands Andy Street. Many, like me, are Aston Villa supporters. Few are professors or social scientists but, rather amazingly, in the same *patrol* in my school Scout troop (and there were four school Scout troops, with four patrols in each), in the space of five years, were the sociologist and research methods guru Professor Nigel Gilbert (he was my patrol leader), and pro- fessor of history and public policy at the University of Cambridge Simon Szreter; I was his patrol leader!

Three varieties of qualitative inquiry over the years

I knew the Boys for a couple of years before I formally embarked on 'researching' them. I lived on their patch. I played for the local soccer teams, often with some of their older brothers (later with some of them). I drank in one of the local pubs. I was, initially, a volunteer at the nearby 'adventure playground', which was also often referred to as 'the Rec', as it was on the edge of the recreation ground, or as the 'youth club'. So even before I started my research, I had some knowledge and understanding of 'the Boys' – the 'rec Boys', as they were known. Indeed, it was only because of the existing relationships I had with them that I contemplated and broached with them the idea of a research study focusing in on their criminal behaviour and experience of the criminal justice system – policing, the courts and custody. For some of the Boys, their entry point to that system had been non-school attendance, for which they were prosecuted. But non-attendance at school had also led to 'hanging around' all day, which produced early engagement in both instrumental and expressive delinquency – raising money through shoplifting and burglary, stealing cars and wrecking bus shelters and telephone boxes 'for fun' (see Williamson 1978). On one occasion, two of them even hijacked a double-decker bus, when the driver left the engine running while he stepped out to make a phone call (from a telephone box); the two boys spotted the opportunity to 'have a laugh', though the terrified passengers were not so sure – and the boys were each sentenced to three months in Detention Centre for their ten minutes of fun!

For the research study, I spent the best part of the next two years just hanging around with the Boys. Rarely did a day go by without me spending some time with them. I knew their routines and it was usually easy to find them, on the street corner, up at the recreation ground, in the woods and, increasingly, in the pub. I associated with them in all these settings and accumulated a sense of what made them tick and what motivated their behaviour. I went to court with them and visited them in various forms of custody.[35] On the weekends, I went to town with them. On occasions, I was invited into their homes. This was 'participant observation' *par excellence*; no part of their lives was concealed from me, though I did not take part in everything they did. But the Boys (or at least most of them) came to trust me and seemed quite happy to reveal things to me, either of their own volition or in response to my insatiable curiosity. As I have often quipped, my own life was

35 They had to send me a 'VO' (Visiting Order) and I often went with their mothers, though sometimes on my own. In the former case, it was easier to pretend I was 'with' their mother, my arm dangling around her shoulder, rather than explain that I was a university postgraduate research student, given all the questions that might invite. Predictably, as a result, I was associated with the family and treated accordingly – sometimes abusively, much more often with 'casual' derogatory remarks, and routinely with petty actions (instructions, delays, interruptions) to convey strongly where power resided in the institution. It was an interesting, if sometimes unpleasant, experience and a striking contrast to the way I was treated, many years later, when I visited Young Offender Institutions, Secure Training Centres and local authority secure children's homes as a board member of the Youth Justice Board, with my Home Office pass that accorded me 'unrestricted but accompanied' access to all areas.

quite opposite to theirs and this played out in my own behaviour. I was the honest man amongst thieves, I was the peaceful person in a violent culture, and I *never* accepted stolen property but *always* asked the questions.

Though a large group of them visited me in Birmingham each year every December, after I left Milltown in 1979, my contact with them steadily diminished, though I did stay in touch with Marty, Danny, Ted and Jerry, visiting them from time to time. Twenty years later, after a consultation with Danny in the autumn of 1999, I renewed contact with the Boys for reasons to do with sociological theory, policy considerations and human interest. Ulrich Beck (1992) had established the concept of 'risk society', the 'new Labour' government was concerned about 'social exclusion' and young people who were 'NEET' (not in employment, education or training), and I – as a 'youth policy' adviser to various governments on issues including education, vocational training, substance misuse and crime – wondered what had happened to the Milltown Boys. With a small grant from the National Lottery Charities Board to consider the 'health' of the Milltown Boys in middle age, I spent a year getting in touch with 30 of them in order to talk to them about the pathways they had taken over the previous 20 years. My semi-structured tape-recorded interviews during the year 2000 yielded 500,000 words of transcript, on all facets of their lives and how their life course had unfolded over the preceding years.

For a third round of contact and communication, nearly 50 years after first meeting the Boys, there were serious questions about an appropriate 'methodology'. Clearly, participant observation was no longer an option, although there was the possibility of joining in some of their routine social events. I was aware that it might not be so easy to find the Boys in the pubs; the past decade has – as we shall hear from the Boys themselves – decimated the number of pubs in Milltown. I was unsure whether semi-structured interviews would work this time, leaning towards more opportunistic and spontaneous exchanges of experiences and perspectives, and – something that had not been an option previously – social media. The Covid-19 crisis, however, presented an unexpected and different opportunity to forge contact with the Boys and to request an online interview. As a result, during the three months of the first lockdown and just afterwards, 12 of the Boys were formally interviewed for the bulk of the material in this book. So, as Table 3.1 indicates, the

TABLE 3.1 Different approaches to data collection on The Milltown Boys

1973–1978
Participant observation: on the street, in court, in custody

1999–2004
Extended interviews lasting hours and covering 'everything'

2017–2020
Phone calls/social media communication, and online research interviews

research dimension of my relationship with the Boys has taken different forms over the years, adapting to circumstances and seizing possibilities.

Tentative steps

The first thing I had to do was to secure institutional ethical approval for a follow-up study of the Boys. Ethics had hardly even been an issue before. In the 1970s, it was remotely associated with medical ethics and rarely a formal consideration within the social sciences. At the turn of the millennium, it was still not prominent in social research, though there was some interest in ethical responsibility (notably around confidentiality and consent) and there were light-touch expectations and procedures at play. By 2020, ethics were firmly embedded within any research process, particularly if it carried some level of risk, or involved vulnerable groups, sensitive issues or risky situations. This was therefore a necessary, though for me a somewhat bizarre, step of the journey. On the one side, I was chair of the Faculty Research Ethics Committee, so I was unsure quite how to process my own application. On the other side, there was the rather unusual, if not unique, fact that I was hardly venturing out to find a sample and secure consent from prospective respondents. Indeed, I had already spent a number of years both talking through, with some of the Boys, the idea of further research,[36] and reacting to *their* not infrequent suggestion, certainly from some of them, that 'it's time for you to write another book'. When I just dropped by to see Matt in the autumn of 2019, after I had made contact out of concern because of his life-threatening illness, he said that he knew I would "probably be showing up soon, because *another* twenty years have gone by". I had only seen him one other time (when I visited him in prison in 2007) in the intervening years. At that point, some months after the visit, in April, he sent me a letter outlining all his new plans on his release:

> Hello Howard how's things hope you and your family are happy and in good health please tell them an old friend said hello and hopes there alright and give them my best. Well mate sorry I haven't wrote back until now but I been trying to sort out a few things you see me and a friend are going to open a salon in Milltown, where both doing a barbering course and are close to

36 The first of 'the Boys', though not one who featured in my 2004 book, to turn 60 did so in June 2019. Though he still mixed with the 'catholic' Boys – Tony, Spaceman, Gary, Kelvin, Jamie, Gordon and others – he had not lived in Milltown for many years, had a professional job, and was a very reflective conversationalist. In late summer 2019, I went to his house and tape-recorded a chat with him about the general context of the Boys' histories and current circumstances, and what he thought about my idea of doing further research on and with them. He had extricated himself from the crazy young adult years of the Boys following being charged with affray, alongside Gary and Kelvin. That experience had terrified him and he had determined to avoid any further brushes with the law and possible conviction and imprisonment. Though he still drank heavily, he was otherwise quite a health fanatic, on account of a childhood illness that had nearly killed him. The material from this interview has *not* been included in this book.

passing it, it's only N.V.Q level two but it means im a barber and that's something no one can take away, we have got to apply for some grants from all kinds of people, so if you can help us in anyway we would be very happy for any kind of help because he's out next Month and im not out until 9-8-07 so he will look for some wear for a salon we have already got a grant for £5.000 and got to pay £140 a Month back, so it will be good if I get my tag I have applied for it now the thing is I wasn't going to apply for it but Zelda my daughter wants me out and she said I can go and live with her, so with a bit of luck I could be out this Month, if not I'll be able to work in the salon on stage two that means when I finish stage one which I starts on Monday for a Month or two I can get a job on stage two and get paid, so by the time he gets the salon started I should be on stage two, I don't think I will be rich but it will help make a living and if that can keep me out of prison that's all good, can't think of anything else to talk about so all the best from an old friend to a good Mate thanks for all you've done and for being there for all of us Thanks,
    Matt

I was not able to help Matt in the way I had supported Spaceman. The salon plan never worked out as Matt had hoped (see Chapter 5), and it was well over ten years before I saw Matt again.

Having secured ethics approval from the University (with the help of the Research Governance Officer, who had translated my rather relaxed application form into 'more formal' language), and had my 'Information Sheet' and 'Consent Form' accepted, I was now – in January 2020 – in a position to request a formal research interview with the Boys. Before I did so, however (as noted above), Ted had actually *requested* to be interviewed, arguing that from his side he could gather some thoughts as to what somebody might say at his funeral (which would, according to his prognosis, probably be within the next three years), while from my side it could be material for 'another book' and he would be quite happy for me to "ask anything you like". That, then, was technically my first 'research interview' despite the fact that, although I had cleared the ground to proceed from a research ethics point of view, I was still in the process of exploring the feasibility of doing a further study and considering a range of issues.

Getting the Boys' consent and the interviews done

Driving back with Danny from another visit to Ted's (a few weeks after my research interview with him), I asked Danny if he would mind being interviewed. He said it would be "no problem, whenever you're ready". But the key individual for me was Gary. After considerable reticence about another study on the part of at least some of the Boys, it had been at Gary's son's funeral that there appeared to be some change of mind and reasonably strong consensus that I should think seriously about writing another book. That was when I really did start thinking *seriously* about doing so. But I needed to be sure that Gary would be comfortable about it. It was only in April 2020 that I summoned up the courage to ask him directly about it. Without hesitation, he said it was fine. He dismissed the request as a stupid question and said that, anyway, *he* had a lot to say! I told him how relieved I was; in the absence of a green light from Gary, I would have stopped this research in its tracks. I determined to dedicate the book to Adrian, so long as Gary was happy for me to do so.[37]

By April 2020, however, the UK was already four weeks into the Covid-19 lockdown. And this revealed the Boys' abject knowledge of the use of technology. I had been compelled to embark on a sharp learning curve (my own knowledge was rudimentary in early March), but they had no idea whatsoever what to do. Like me only weeks before, when I mentioned WhatsApp, Zoom, Hangouts, Teams, Messenger and other social media communication platforms, they had no idea what I was talking about. Danny had never sent a text message until January 2020, when we were arranging to visit Ted. Once Gary had, during a phone call, agreed both to the research overall and to be interviewed, he had to check how he might do it with his daughter, Simone:

> What platform do you want to use for video chat on Friday? Just so I can ask my daughter to help me out with set up ☺ Gary

Others of the Boys had neither the confidence nor the equipment to proceed, other than their mobile phones. Mark described his phone as "a Doctor Who phone", meaning its antiquity not futuristic character. He said I would have to link up with him on his wife Veronica's phone, through WhatsApp, "but don't ask me how you do that, I've never even sent a text message"! But eventually, one way and another, by the end of July 2020, I had managed to interview a dozen of the Boys for an hour or more, and in the process discovered quite a lot about what had happened to most of the others who had featured in *The Milltown Boys Revisited*.

Once I got cracking on the 'research interviews', I used a very loose framework of topics to guide the conversation (see Table 3.2). The encounter was set up in many different ways. Jamie suggested that the best time for an interview was early on a Saturday afternoon, "because that's when I'd normally be in the bookies". Matt retreated to his son's bedroom, whom he was visiting when I called. Paul cancelled one agreed time and rescheduled it on his terms, once he'd had a few drinks to pluck up the confidence to talk. Gary planned to use his sister's office, which was just over the road from his flat, and downloaded Zoom for the occasion but it didn't work and we reverted to a phone call. Vic talked to me from a corner of Ted's living room; Ted was getting comfortably stoned in another corner. When Vic turned his phone camera towards Ted to show me Ted was there, he mumbled

---

37 When I broached this with Gary, he said he would be 'honoured' if I was to dedicate the book to Adrian. After I ended the call, he immediately rang his ex-wife Amelia, Adrian's mother, to tell her, and then he called me straight back; she was equally delighted at, and equally touched by the idea. 'No problem, H', Gary said.

almost incoherently that Vic "should do one of those interviews like I done with you", clearly unaware that was exactly what I was doing at that very moment! Danny called me from his phone, when he had some 'free' time away from his grandson; we snatched at the issues and I kept a record of where we had got to, so that we didn't run over the same ground. I used the final segment to secure from Danny a more profound retrospective on the Boys and on our own rather unexpected and special relationship throughout our lives. Spaceman's hearing problems proved difficult but we worked out a way, even if a number of issues had to be repeated. Indeed, I worked out a way with most of the Boys, one way or another! It was not, however, plain sailing even then. I got Jerry's phone number and called him, but – as in 2000 – he was reticent about being 'interviewed', but even more so. These days, he said, he kept himself to himself and didn't want to talk. I was, of course, disappointed. Jerry – alongside Danny, Ted, Marty and Pete – had been at the heart of my original research. But, for perfectly understandable reasons, which I completely respect and do not wish to reveal, he had no wish to have his personal circumstances projected into the public domain once again.

There were different issues in relation to Pete. I had stumbled across a phone number in some old notes and called, completely expecting the line to now be dead or to get an answerphone message. Instead, Pete answered. We talked, immediately, for well over an hour, during which time Pete said that my call had made him 'feel a bit jelly-like' – "it's knocked me sideways, like a bolt out of the blue". I told him that it had been quite a surprise to me, when he answered the phone; his rejoinder was that "at least *you* were prepared". He said he had become almost a complete recluse and suffered profoundly from depression. He needed time to digest our conversation. We agreed a formal 'research interview' for the following day (a Saturday, at 09.30, when his partner Barry would still be sleeping) but, within hours, Pete had sent me a text message (in capital letters), saying he did not feel able to go ahead and would send me an email to explain. At 05.22 the following morning, he did, and it had a lovely tone. Here it is, in abbreviated form:

> Hi Howard, it really was good to talk to you yesterday ... And to hear some news about the people from Milltown.
> Sorry no phone call, I'm afraid it sent my anxiety through the roof.
> I would like to help you in any way I am able, but I find direct communication quite difficult.
> I was wondering if you could put your questions by email?
> I can't guarantee to answer the questions, or how long it will take to answer, but I will do my best.
> Best wishes,
> Pete

I spent some hours elaborating on the Topic Guide I had been using in my interviews with the Boys (see below), adding many supplementary questions and pointing out that

They have not so much been questions but themes around which we have pursued a conversation, but I will try to turn them into questions and hope that you may find the time and spirit to address them as fully or thinly as you can and wish to do so.

The questions were still, unfortunately, too overwhelming. Regrettably, and clearly after much deliberation, Pete sent me another message:

Hi Howard,
I'm really sorry but I won't be able to help on this project.
I find reminiscing really hard to do.
Again I'm very sorry.
All the best for the future,
Pete

I wrote back saying that I fully understood and respected his decision although I noted that 'from a professional position' I thought his perspective was particularly special and would have added a distinctive angle on the material for the book. I was, naturally, deeply disappointed but I did not relay that to him; paradoxically, Pete has found escape and happiness through his homosexuality but has always struggled to deal with his roots. Even at the age of 22, when the BBC recorded 'Five Years', questions were asked in some reviews whether he really could be from Milltown because he was so articulate; after some years living in London and inhabiting the gay scene there, he had already lost his Milltown accent. Yet only a few years earlier, in part because he was tall and loud, he had been portrayed (by prosecuting solicitors) or assumed (by the police and magistrates) to be one of the ringleaders amongst the Boys and, at the youngest possible age (14), he had served a custodial

TABLE 3.2 Topic Guide – The Milltown Boys at 60

General update – what's been happening in the past 20 years?
Employment/benefits
Health
Relationships
Children/grandchildren
Crime
Housing
Politics – austerity; Brexit; Covid-19
Religion/faith
Leisure time – domestic; holidays; hobbies
Networks and friends
Keeping contact with the Boys
Looking back and early thoughts about me
General overview

sentence in Detention Centre for persistent offending. He certainly had the image of being one of the roughest and toughest of the Boys. Just a few years later, he came out as gay and left the estate for good.

I recount this part of Pete's story here simply to point out that while renewed contact with the Milltown Boys has been quite remarkable in some ways, it has not been without its challenges and setbacks. Even the best of relationships forged in previous years, as with both Jerry and Pete, were not sufficient to encourage their participation in this study. For very different reasons, they declined, courteously and warmly, not wishing to take part but also still not wishing to lose touch. I have respected and appreciated that.

Those I did manage to interview considered the issues outlined in Table 3.2, many of which were triggered in response to the first open question: 'tell me what's been happening to you over the past 20 years?' Some emphasised their employment trajectories on either side of the law. Some talked first about their families and their relationships, especially their (usually) young grandchildren. Others focused on health issues that had affected them. Few mentioned any of the other topics without some prompting and probing. It was a relaxed, generally warm, and always enjoyable encounter, despite the technological obstructions. There was, inevitably, some nostalgia and reminiscing but that in itself provided me with the opportunity to use it as a launch pad to explore what had happened since. We did not go over too much old ground, but it generally did not feel like 20 years since we had spoken to each other.

PART II

4

ORIGINS AND DESTINATIONS

Origins and Destinations is the title of a classic book on social mobility by Halsey[38] *et al.* (1980); it was preoccupied with the role of social class in education, and the impact of education on social class, in terms of the occupational destinations of those from different class backgrounds. It was criticised for having focused only on men (as, indeed, this study might be, too), but it did seem to show the modest impact of the British educational system on the social class structure of Britain. Despite the supposed establishment of 'equality of educational opportunity', the social reproduction of class position has proved remarkably stubborn. Successive Prime Ministers from across the political spectrum have consistently and repeatedly proclaimed that education, through 'meritocracy',[39] is the key to reaching destinations that are 'better' and 'higher' than the circumstances, the origins, where individuals started their lives. Yet research tells us, equally consistently, that it is not schools (or universities), but differences in home environments, and particularly the time that parents can give to their children, that facilitate or obstruct equality of opportunity (see Bukodi and Goldthorpe 2018).

38 The late A.H. Halsey (1923–2014) – 'Chelly' to those who knew him – was a distinguished professor of Social and Administrative Studies at the University of Oxford. He was actually the reason I left Milltown in 1979. He appointed me as Research Officer on a major research project evaluating the impact of the Youth Opportunities Programme (see Jones *et al.* 1982). I had no desire to leave Milltown, but colleagues saw the post advertised and suggested it was 'made for me'. I had no expectation of getting the job, but I applied and was successful. As a result, I moved from Milltown to Birmingham, where the fieldwork was to be done, in April 1979. Chelly Halsey's autobiography, *No Discouragement*, is published by Macmillan (1996).

39 Meritocracy, though usually assumed to be a 'good thing', has had its critics, most notably in Michael Young's (1958) dystopian satire *The Rise of the Meritocracy*, in which those who reach the top have absolute belief in their right to be there and those at the bottom have no indigenous champions for their cause and plight and, as a result, sink into a sense of abject despondency and failure.

This evidence should be both good news and bad news for the Milltown Boys. It is good news in the sense that educational achievement, of which the Boys accrued very little, may not anyway have made much difference. It is bad news because purposeful home environments and parental interest, that might have made a difference, were also largely absent for the Boys, who spent most of their time left to their own devices 'somewhere else'. Individual stories do not, of course, necessarily corroborate the statistical evidence but they can convey the nuances at play on the journey from particular origins to what are still, for the Boys, not quite yet final destinations.

None of the Boys had any dramatic 'teenage dreams', or what are sometimes referred to in academic and policy environments as 'unrealistic aspirations', as *The Milltown Boys Revisited* (p.40) suggests:

> The teenage dreams of the Milltown Boys were, inevitably, heavily circumscribed by the narrow occupational and social culture of their neighbourhood. Fathers and older brothers worked on building sites and in factories, and drank down the local pub. No wonder this was also what they expected to do. Given their limited qualifications and the added disadvantage of their juvenile criminal records (and early custodial experiences for some within the adult criminal justice system), it is not surprising the Boys' teenage dreams were largely framed by the twin philosophies of short-termism and entrenched fatalism. Live for today, they argued, for there is little personal capacity to influence the future – an approach to their lives established in their mid-teens, which became more strongly reinforced as the Boys entered early adulthood.

The observation in *The Milltown Boys Revisited* that some of the Boys have been quite successful, if not exactly flourished, should therefore be considered a significant celebration of success. The story of the Milltown Boys, up to the age of 40, was by no means just a commiseration with failure, on account of childhood origins giving way to adult lives in the 'precariat' (see Standing 2011) at the bottom end of the labour market or outside of it, and in the deviant cultures of drugs and crime, even if this was the story for a significant number of them. About a third of them, through different combinations of luck and judgement, have done quite well.

Gary phoned me during the Covid-19 crisis (on 20 April 2020) to ask for Ted's phone number; he had heard that Ted was ill and wanted to get in touch with him, though they had not been in contact for some years. In the conversation on the phone, Gary talked at length about origins and destinations. He was, simultaneously, equally critical of those of the Boys who now sometimes denied or glossed over their starting points in life (like Tony and Gordon) and those who had remained, as he put it, 'stuck' in their roots. In relation to the latter group (not just the hard men, like Ted, Vic, Danny and Matt, but others like Paul, Mack and Colin – essentially those who became *The Fountain* Boys after some years in *The Wayfarer* (until it closed), though *The Fountain* pub has now also closed and been converted into luxury apartments – Gary spoke proudly: "when I was a kid, I ran with those boys". They had been the closest members of his peer group, and he still loved them dearly. Indeed, he had recently bumped into Paul, who had greeted him like a long-lost friend, which is in fact exactly what he was – for a long time, not part of Gary's adult friendship circle, having been lost to drugs, drink and crime. This was, sadly, the story for quite a number of the Boys. Even Danny who, until quite recently, was one of *The Fountain* Boys, commented that too many of those Boys, when he saw them in the street, were just looking for a handout: 'help me out with a fiver, Danny; give me a tenner'. But he had never for a moment thought he himself would end up like that; he insisted he had always been too methodical and careful with his offending. It had never become chaotic, or desperate, as it had with some of the Boys. Mark said pointedly that too many of the Boys were now "ravaged by drugs", noting that apart from some glue-sniffing "all I've ever done is drink, and I don't even do much of that now". He was proud to have always worked, yet attributed his particular pathway in life to the fact that his father helped him to join the working-men's social club long before he was legally old enough to drink, where he then "followed in the footsteps of the older men, playing old men's games like Dom and Crib", and so avoiding the deviant and addictive cultures of the pubs, notably *The Wayfarer* and then *The Fountain*: "those Boys went their way, whereas I had the club". Mark's perspective is remarkably in tune with Phil Cohen's (1997) concepts of 'apprenticeship' and 'inheritance' in his analysis of the way working-class sons follow in the footsteps of their fathers. It was not something that featured so prominently in the lives of many of the other Milltown Boys.

Like Mark, Gary had attended the comprehensive school but he had ended up in what Mark called the 'culture of *The Wayfarer*', that in his view had set those Boys who gathered there on the wrong path. How then had Gary avoided a lifetime of offending and sometimes also dependency on drink and drugs? Gary said that the 'work ethic', instilled in him by his father ("we always had food on the table; we never had to scrape around") had saved him from that fate. I was still slightly perplexed and asked Gary how he had moved from that friendship group to becoming in effect, as a young adult, one of the 'catholic' Boys (mixing with Spaceman, Tony, Kelvin, Jamie, Gordon and Derek and sometimes involving Marty). He said it was the simple fact of getting banned from *The Wayfarer*. Caught throwing skittles balls at beer bottles in the skittle alley, Gary, Marty and Alex were – at the age of 17! – banned from the pub. Alex elected to try to get a drink in *The Carpenter's Arms* at the top of the estate, while Marty, who had attended the catholic school (erratically[40]) though his offending profile was very different from most

40 Marty's case is a classic example of inconsistent child-rearing. He lived, most of the time with his grandmother, Ruby. Ruby's boyfriend, Jack, was a labourer who drank heavily. He was often violent. If he discovered that Marty had been missing school, which was often the case, he would physically beat him. Yet the following day he would tell Marty he would not be going to school because he had to stay in for the coalman to make a delivery, or for some other reason. Ruby was a cleaner at *The Wayfarer*; she did not intervene – she usually simply smiled and said rather sadly that it was 'just the way it is'. Jack was the man of the house, and she, Marty and his brother Daniel had to do

of the 'catholic' Boys, persuaded Gary to join up with the 'catholic' Boys in *The Centurion*, to the west of the estate. He therefore attributed his 'destination', towards a fairly successful retirement having worked hard all of his life, not only to his family background but to that moment of chance. At heart, he was still a steadfast Milltown Boy, immensely proud of his roots, background and upbringing, but also still excited and enthusiastic about discovering new worlds and new people. Locked down for four weeks during the Covid-19 crisis, he was already missing working in London, where every day was different, though he was now looking forward to a walk through the woods adjacent to Milltown, where he had spent a lot of his younger teenage days sniffing glue and fighting by the river with the Fairfield Boys. He had not been down there for years. Gary was completely rooted in Milltown, but able to embrace the wider world. Other Boys who had also embraced the wider world (notably Tony and Gordon, arguably Shaun too, and also, in a very different way, Pete, who cut himself off from Milltown completely at the age of 16) were reticent about talking about their origins in Milltown, even if they did not disown their roots absolutely, and Gary felt that they should hold their heads high about where they had come from. Equally, though, Gary was sad that too many of the Boys from his childhood days (certainly Danny, possibly more than any of them, Mack, Colin, Paul and Mark, probably also Tommy, Denny and Mal and, to a significantly lesser extent, Jerry, Ryan and Trevor) celebrated their Milltown roots because they had never really gone anywhere else; Milltown had been their origins and has remained their destination.

---

as they were told or suffer the consequences. Marty stayed away from Jack as much as he possibly could; a smack round the head, 'for nothing', was the best he could expect if they passed each other in the house.

5

EMPLOYMENT

The employment pathways of the Milltown Boys have been strikingly diverse. Whether or not these should be referred to as 'careers' is debatable, for many routes were significantly influenced by extraneous episodes and events. The Boys rarely had a plan, but some did seize opportunities when they presented themselves. Most of the Boys have remained, one way and another, in manual work, though even there a diversity of activity has been followed. Only a few have worked for most of their lives in 'white collar' professional occupations, and only Jamie made the dramatic transition, shortly before he turned 40, from hard manual labour (working on building sites and laying tarmac) to an 'office job' (running the post room for an insurance company). At the time he saw this as no more than a temporary move, to tide him over Christmas and have the money to buy presents for the kids, but he is still there, maintaining that while more senior people had been made redundant as services were automated, his roles had been extended because he was 'cheap'! Clearly, other attractions of the job – working with women, holiday pay, flexitime, free coffee, being indoors and having a shower *before* he went to work (see *The Milltown Boys Revisited*, pp.62–63) – outweighed what he always considered to be terrible pay, certainly compared to laying tarmac. When I talked with Jamie, in April 2020, he was still celebrating his lucky break at having the job he has; even though he was working from home because of lockdown, he was "popping into the building" every day to turn on the taps and let the water run through. That at least broke up the monotony of the day! Bizarrely, when job cuts and restructuring were being carried out, some four years ago, Jamie was half-hoping to be made redundant and he recognised the irony that, on that occasion, in contrast to his own cautious and experimental approach to a new kind of work suggested by a neighbour (in November 1996), it was the company that had suggested he tried his proposed new role on a temporary basis:

Well, obviously with email and that, there's less and less to do in a Post Room. We'd steadily gone down from five or six people to just me. And then the company had started to lay other people off and I was waiting for my turn to come. But they kept getting rid of my bosses, and they kept asking me to take on more and more of their responsibilities. I'm only little old Jamie with two CSEs and they'd been to uni. I didn't really want to do these things.... I was sort of saying No but not actually saying No because I wanted them to make me redundant. And I was a bit nervous, to tell you the truth. I wasn't sure I could do it. But then I thought, what have you got to lose? Give it a try. They asked me to give it a go for a couple of weeks. And that two weeks has lasted another four years. The company has been taken over, but I was TUPE'd.[41] So, all in all, I've been with this company now for nearly 25 years. Not bad for a job that was going to tide me over Christmas! I'm still not that confident with the I.T. side of things, and I have to set up all the equipment, but I've got by.

Having said all of that, retirement crosses my mind every single day, and I'd snap their hands off if they offered it to me.

Jamie is relaxed about contemplating retirement because his finances are secure. He has a comfortable occupational pension to look forward to, his own house is fully paid for, and he noted that one of the best things that he'd ever done was to buy his parents' house in Milltown (see Chapter 10), which he described as "my safety-net for the future".

Two of the Boys have been astonishingly successful in their working lives. Tony worked for one company until he was in his 50s, as he was promoted to a senior managerial position. The company was taken over and, about a year later (around 2007), realising he "wasn't happy" in the new structure and despite being offered an even better job, he joined another supply chain company as a partner, making good use of many of the contacts he had forged in his previous job:

I took a gamble by leaving a company that I'd worked for all of my life to join a failing firm, but I just knew it had loads of potential. It had been a good company but it had become a weak business because it had lost a few major clients and didn't seem able to embrace new challenges. And we've done fantastically well. My old company sold to industry tools and equipment. We sell to industry electronic components. So the product is different, but the customer base is the same.

There was no conflict of interests. I could not have left my old company and gone to work for a competitor, because they'd been good to me all my life. With this company, I could talk to all my old contacts about a new

41 Transfer of Undertakings and Protection of Employment (TUPE) – this is when individuals transfer from one company to another: the intention is to preserve the terms and conditions of their employment, at least for some period of time.

product, a different product. Our clients are predominantly manufacturing businesses – big names: Siemens, Rolls Royce, AstraZeneca, Unilever, Nestlé, JCB, General Motors. Our main sectors are pharmaceutical, automotive, food and beverage, energy – all big household names that you would know. We're not that big. We operate in a radius of about 50 miles, so we deal with divisions of those companies. We're not worldwide; I wish we were! We're on target this year for a turnover of about six million. And yes, I own the company, 50/50 with my business partner. Split down the middle.

Tony was described in *The Milltown Boys Revisited* (p.49) as having "done very well for himself", having started in a temporary job with the tools and equipment company as a stock control clerk in 1977. That, today, would be a dramatic understatement!

Gordon was already doing very well in 2000 and has continued with his varied entrepreneurial activities as well as working, from time to time, as a business consultant dealing with organisational change. He contemplates stopping work 'quite soon' though currently he combines a variety of legitimate business interests and consultancy work. He recently ended a year's consultancy on HR issues for a large fish-exporting company, with plans to go travelling once again. His wife Michaela still owns her hairdressing salons, and they still have their properties. Gordon, having been made redundant a few years ago, was not planning to 'work' (as an employee, or for somebody else) again, but the consultancy work he was asked to do constituted, as he put it, "an offer I couldn't refuse". The travelling has had to be put on hold.

But these professional and entrepreneurial careers were the exceptions. Most of the Boys on the right side of the law ticked along in manual occupations. The most consistently employed of that group (namely those positioned in between the few more successful of them and those existing on the other side of legitimate employment) were those working in state or state-related sectors, such as the railways or the Post Office. Mark, indeed, after nearly 20 years working on the railways, was made redundant and, after a year in the steelworks (where he found attention to health and safety conspicuous mainly by its absence in comparison with his experience on the railways, "so I got out"), became a postman. He literally adores the job, noting the striking contrast between his consummate honesty these days and his teenage 'thieving' years[42]:

> I love my job…. I am as honest as they come, How, you've got to be. See, when it happens – you know, taking from Christmas and birthday cards, special deliveries, taking *from children* – everyone looks at the postman anyway, even if it could've been somebody else….

---

42 Jerry had also noted, in *The Milltown Boys Revisited* (p.87), that being a postman demanded inherent honesty, describing how he had recently returned an expensive watch he had found in the street, "whereas I suppose twenty years ago I would have been wearing it"!

Yeah, I love my job. Even with all the things I done when I was younger, it's never entered my head. I used to do a round up Highbroughton [a really desirable village, geographically not far from Milltown but in terms of social class and property prices, light years away] and this package had come open and it was all these money vouchers, so I picked the ones that had fell out from off the floor. So anyway, I knocked the door and explained, and she said 'don't worry'. As it happened, it was all there, about £1,000 in vouchers, so there wasn't a problem, but I was worried for a moment. But she said 'don't worry, I trust you'. Yeah, they trust me.

Whatever round I've been on, they love me. I just get on great with people. When I was up Highbroughton they'd give me the codes to their gates and the locks on their sheds, so I could leave parcels.... When you think we used to nick all their apples! I remember, when I was a kid, we went up there, to the shop – it was obviously owned by different people then – and we robbed the place blind. We went through the birds' nests up there and they had nothing left, you know what I mean!

But it was great up there, a great round. When I had to leave, because the rounds go on seniority and I had to go elsewhere, the village council got together and wrote a letter saying they wanted me to stay. But I had to move on.

I asked Mark what constituted a 'good' round, as a postman. On the one hand, he said, it was where the dogs were under control and, on the other, where you got more appreciation and better tips. He said he would not want to be a postman in Milltown again, though this was where he had started:

Don't get me wrong. I love Milltown. I've lived here all my life, haven't I? But there's the dog situation. It's not so bad now, because not so many let their dogs roam the streets, but it's still a bit of a shit hole, half the place, How, everybody knows that. I love the place, I'd never move out of here, but it's still a shit hole. Even without the dogs, when I used to deliver up here, everybody would know you and want you to stop and have a chat and a cup of tea – you'd never get your round finished! It'd take you forever.

At Christmas time, you'd probably get tips from more people in Milltown than you would up Highbroughton, because there's some tight-fisted arseholes up there – you know, How, there's good and bad in all walks of life – but the good ones are really generous. When I was up there, I had a better wine cellar than fucking Dom Kimaki, and I don't even drink the bleeding stuff! People are generous to us if you look after them over the year. So, yeah, I'm really enjoying the job, even after 17 years. It's a great job. You meet different people all the time. It's not as easy as a lot of people think, but it's very rewarding. You get to know people. You see their kids grow up. You build up a rapport with them. You win their trust. You meet some real characters. There's one old fella, he's a multi-millionaire, who's into horses. I think he owns a few. I'd get his papers from the shop – the *Financial Times*, the *Racing Post* – and take them along to him. He'd always offer you a tenner or £20 – 'have a drink on me' – and at Christmas time, he'd give you a ton (£100). Such down to earth people for all their money. Not a bit of snobbery about them. One of them was a barrister. I nearly asked him to defend Veronica [see below] but at the end of the day it wasn't his field of law, but I think if I had asked him, he would have helped to find someone to do it.

Jerry continued working as a postman until he was invalided out at the age of 52, after an unsuccessful operation on his feet. The Post Office had requested a 'work capability assessment' which was conducted privately and Jerry was declared unfit for work. On that account, he had his pension entitlement dramatically brought forward. Shortly after retiring, it was suggested that he might still be eligible for some state benefits. He made inquiries and was subjected to another work capability assessment by Job Centre Plus (Department of Work and Pensions [DWP]). Though conducted by the same company, which had the national contract for this work with the DWP, this time he was declared fit for work. He told them where to stuff the small amount to which he might have been entitled and hobbled away. Technically, Jerry still works, at least in the sense that he receives an attendance allowance as the designated carer for his daughter, Rachael, who has profound physical and learning disabilities.

Matt has also retired, at least in a way. When he served time in prison in his 40s, he had trained as a hairdresser inside and, on release, had hoped there might be something for him in that line of work (see his letter to me, above), but instead he continued doing menial and manual jobs here and there, though sometimes these were, to him, quite inspiring and appealing, such as working on the window display for some notable retail fashion outlets in London, including Jimmy Choo. But he lost that job when he was sent to prison once again for 18 weeks, at the age of 57, for breaching a restraining order and subsequently he had further confrontations with the police. He thought he might have got his cleaning job back but decided, as he put it, to 'self-section' himself to avoid more brushes with the law and the risk of further imprisonment – in effect, then, cutting himself off from the world, except for his family. As a result, he lives alone and does not work, venturing out only to meet his youngest son from school or to spend time with his grandchildren. Matt described his 'working life', if it could be called that, as "a sequence of squandered opportunities", on both sides of the law, though it was also interesting that he noted, "You know, it's funny, How, it seems the worse I'm paid, the happier I am":

When you're breaking the law, you're usually on your own, or just with a few others and you don't want to tell anybody about it. It can be really lonely. Whereas when you're in a cleaning team, you're with loads of people and you can have a laugh and you can tell people about what you do. You know, I can tell everybody about the chandeliers at Jimmy Choo.

See I was working for this cleaning company and I did all the windows in these big office blocks. And I was so good… you mustn't leave any streaks, you have to do it in one stroke. They started calling me The Glass Man. And they sent me to London. I cleaned the glass at Hugo Boss and Jimmy Choo. They've got these massive chandeliers and they're worth a fortune. You've got to take a lot of care. And I was brilliant at it. I've got loads of photos of my work. Everybody said I was the best.

But then I got sent to prison and after I come out I never had nowhere to live. I was homeless for a bit – just floor space in a hostel when I didn't have any other places to go. It was torture. I wasn't really thinking about work. And then I got this flat in sheltered housing. I could've gone back to work but the flat would have taken all my wages. I suppose I could've done cash in hand but, no, I decided to give up work and concentrate on my boy.

Pete, in his younger days, had done spells as a cashier in petrol stations but, for a long time now, like Jerry, he is also a designated carer; he has been looking after his partner Barry since 1996 when he was severely injured by a nail through the head in the Atlanta bombing in 1996.[43] Tommy has now retired, after many years as a street cleaner with the council. He, too, is a carer, looking after his wife, following her brain aneurism some years ago.

Ryan is still a council employee, working in the city parks. Others continued to turn their hand at different employment opportunities in the legitimate labour market, working continuously but within different activities. For example, Alex now does 'odd jobs' in the relatively affluent neighbourhood where he lives – "a bit of gardening, a bit of house maintenance, for £15.00 an hour". The upholstery business he joined as a teenager and then inherited from his boss eventually collapsed but by then he was reasonably comfortably off. The most important thing remained having the flexibility to go and watch his beloved Arsenal at every possible opportunity. Trevor continues to fit windows, though he is contemplating retirement, in order to spend more time with his grandchildren. However, it is, ironically, his five grandchildren who keep him working, because he is always trying to respond financially to their demands: "I'm trying to establish some kind of rationing plan, but everyone always breaks whatever we've agreed to". Kelvin was a semi-professional photographer for many years but then switched to fitting kitchens and bathrooms (with tiling as a speciality). This is what he is still doing, self-employed and sub-contracting:

---

43 The Centennial Olympic Park bombing was a pipe bomb attack in Atlanta, Georgia, during the 1996 Summer Olympics. The blast killed one person directly and another later died of a heart attack. A total of 111 people were injured. The back pack that exploded had contained three pipe bombs surrounded by three-inch long (7.6 cm) masonry nails.

When I was trying to find Pete in 1999, a number of the Boys told me they had 'seen him on the telly, at that bombing in America'. I had not really believed this, thinking it must be a case of mistaken identity, but it turned out to be true.

Yeah, I stopped doing photography when it went digital. But I'd also got into tiling, and I was doing photography as well. And when it went digital, I didn't really want to get into that, so I stopped. Plus, I was earning fantastic money from the tiling, so I made more money on a Saturday doing tiling than I did doing wedding photography. Really, I loved both, but something had to give, and it was the photography. I'd had a couple of near misses [with damaged negatives] and I'd had a good run. I hadn't upset anybody by destroying their wedding day, and I just thought it was about time I gave up on it.

I suppose I stopped completely just after you talked to me last like this [2000]. And though I say it myself, I'm fantastic at tiling floors. I'm on my hands and knees all day and it can be very tiring. I get very tired. You know, I'm an old man aching. But I don't want to give up. I love it anyway, but I couldn't afford to retire. I'd like to be in a position where I could retire, but I don't think I could hack sitting down all day.

Anyway, I haven't got any savings, although downsizing on the house will help. But I've never been a saver. I'm a spender, not a saver. I worry about tomorrow – tomorrow! Luckily, things have worked out for me, so far, but on the way, when I've been able to, I've always spent. I just don't plan. I don't see the point. I might not be here. But for now, yeah, I'm going to carry on working.

Apart from one brief spell during the austerity years after 2008, when work was thin on the ground, Kelvin has never been out of work. Others have worked continuously across different employment sectors, doing a bit here and a bit there, sometimes legally, sometimes on the margins of legality, sometimes 'self-employed' (like Denny, who is now a taxi driver, as was Mal until he had a heart operation and had to finish work) and sometimes employed, usually in building maintenance, cleaning or security work.

Vic's story is particularly noteworthy. On disability benefits at the age of 40, having been told he was never likely to work again because of a serious respiratory disease (contracted through the industrial painting he had done for much of his working life), he started to volunteer with a local homelessness charity. Around the age of 50, we bumped into each other in the city centre and he proudly poked me in the chest (nearly sending me flying; he is a big man and had been a serious rugby player when he was a teenager): "you'd be proud of me, How, why didn't you ever tell me that you can get paid for talking to people?" He explained that the charity had taken him on part-time as a support worker, on the grounds that he seemed to have a natural rapport with many of the rough sleepers who turned up for warmth and hot food. This appreciation and recognition restored Vic's sense of self *and* his belief that he might be able to return to 'real work'.[44] And this is what he eventually

44 Some years later, when I found him, or rather his alias, on Facebook, I sent him a message via Messenger: *Vic: how are you? I was told the other day that you are now working on painting ships. Is this so? What happened to the work with the homeless? Hope things are good. Howard.* He replied almost

did, accelerated by some torrid relationship issues, paradoxically resuming the type of industrial painting work (in the boiler rooms of ocean-going ships) that had created his health problems and incapability for work in the first place:

> My nephew's uncle, he was a foreman, and he offered me a job, only for three weeks in a dry dock, in Germany. I can be a grafter if I want and I worked hard. I'm still strong, or I was then. I came home after that, but the boss liked me and he said he might have some more work for me and within a couple of months I was offered a job. I flew out to Dubai, I was on that for about three months and then within about five days of being home again he called me and said pack your bags, you're going again, and so I was on the same ship for another three months. So I done six months on the same ship and it just went from there. After that, I done three world cruises. I've been all over Asia, Australia, the Caribbean, Scandinavia, America. I've been everywhere. Working down in the engine room, all the steelwork down in the engine room. Same as I was doing before, really, but this time I was travelling round the world. I had a good time, met a lot of nice people. I was on the boats for four and a half years, up to about two or three years ago. But I come home, because I was missing my son and then I got a job at home, in a chemical plant, but then I started getting sick and I was struggling to breathe. And they told me I'd got emphysema, so I had to give that up. That's it, I've been on the sick since then.

There remained a small group amongst the Boys who continued to earn a living outside of legal employment, through patently illegal activities (drug dealing, shoplifting) and through gambling. Some weeks things worked out (a win on the horses or the football, some good 'trading'), sometimes not, but the Boys rarely got caught and usually made some £400–500 a week – "not great money", as Danny put it, but enough to get by on. [In February 2020, the average weekly wage in the UK was £512.] These were, however, no longer the halcyon days of drug dealing, when raising a few thousand pounds a week was relatively easily within the realms of possibility. In fact, they talked rather nostalgically of the times when they exploited the festival goers at events like Glastonbury, where they did not even deal drugs but packaged various concoctions of look-alike substances and sold them to gullible "student types, like you, How", as Ted said, grinning. At that time, a 60 pence investment in a bag of sweets could yield hundreds of pounds in dividends! Making money was not the only rationale for some of these activities; it was also to put one over other people. Scamming an extra pack of cigarettes, through removing the actual cigarettes and carefully refilling an empty carton with some other content, and then cunningly exchanging it for a full pack (by buying the same brand,

immediately (15 October 2017): *Yes, I was with the homeless, but all went wrong in my life. A job on the ships came my way. And since then I have travelled around the world. Hope you're OK. Nice to hear from you.*

switching them over and saying they had inadvertently bought the wrong brand), was a victory over shopkeepers they didn't like, though the Boys said they did feel sorry if somebody they knew ended up buying a cigarette packet filled with kitchen roll!

Even though they were not working legitimately, these Boys still invoked the dialogue of 'work', indeed 'entrepreneurship'[45] – earning a living to provide for the family (see below). They often 'worked' in cahoots with one or two business partners, watching out for each other. They continue to weigh up the changing context of risk and reward, assessing, in the case of shoplifting, CCTV systems, security guards, shop assistants and volume of opportunity and, in the case of drug dealing, profit margins and prospective competition. Buying (or stealing) in bulk enables more successful retail distribution; there are now significant numbers of young men ('kids') on bikes in Milltown and elsewhere earning £70 a week through acting as delivery drivers (riders) for relatively small quantities of contraband, cannabis or other produce while simultaneously taking – sometimes literally – a small cut of each delivery for themselves.

Some might ask how it is possible to exist 'successfully' at the margins without attracting attention or suspicion. Those of the Boys operating in this economic sphere usually continue to claim benefits – otherwise they would attract even greater official curiosity as to how they were making a living – and have continued to be adept at 'playing the system' as social security and income support conditions have become more stringent. Receipt of Universal Credit requires applicants to provide evidence of 35 hours of on-line job search a week. One of the Boys persuaded the Job Centre that computers gave him headaches. Others have been getting Disability Living Allowance, latterly Personal Independence Payments (PIPs) for well over a decade, using ruses such as overdoing their levels of anxiety and depression or presenting themselves when required with a stoop and steadied with a walking stick. In the latter example, the individual in question had certainly been confirmed as having arthritis and he had been in receipt of Employment and Support Allowance (ESA), subject to a work capability assessment. The extent to which it impeded his capacity to work had, however, been in doubt. On appeal, however, as reported below (see Chapter 9), he passed the 15 points needed to continue receiving ESA and then applied for an additional PIP, on account of his back problems.[46] Every extra source of income obviously helped, but social security benefits were relatively marginal to the everyday existence and subsistence needs of these Boys:

> I worked hard for that money but I don't touch it. I never see it. It's for the house. It just goes into her account. I don't want the money. I make my own

---

45 For example, when I asked what his children did, Vic told me one of his sons was "an entrepreneur, like Ted's boy; he's learned from Ted's boy, and *he* was following in his father's footsteps" – a rather thinly disguised message that he was involved in buying and selling illegal substances.

46 The detail about these different benefits may be inaccurate, and how they link together, but it is what the Boys said.

money. That goes for the bills, and for the everyday things the kids want, for my daughter and my grandson, and for the shopping. She'll [partner] have it for the shopping one week, and the next week I'll give her a couple of hundred out of my own money. So she can save a bit. She puts 40 or 50 away most fortnights, towards Christmas. I don't want nothing for me. I've got what I want – golf clubs, fishing rods, bikes, infra-red binoculars. I don't need nothing. What I need to keep my life happy I've got. I've got the kids.

The most important thing was the freedom and flexibility to sustain their place and earning power within the illegal economy. Disability allowances that did not require the Boys to work (or show evidence of seeking work) were perfect for the cause because they provided evidence of legitimate income without cramping their style. And yet few of the Boys operating on the wrong side of the law revel in their illegal occupations, maintaining that they have been almost forced into it by the poverty and paucity of legitimate opportunities.[47] As Danny observed:

Don't get me wrong. I don't enjoy this way of life. If somebody sat me down tomorrow and said to me that they can get me £500 a week, I'd do it. I'd do it. I'm not afraid of hard work. But they offer me £300 a week, you know, minimum wage, and I won't do it. Anyway, I don't really have to think about that any more.

I had not seen or talked to Mack since Marty's funeral, six years ago. He launched straight into the impact of the Covid-19 lockdown on his previous lifestyle, which had been going for a pint and a spliff and doing occasional shoplifting (once or twice a week). Instead, he was stuck in the house but, to his surprise, "it's not too bad". I had asked how he was doing for money. He reminded me that he had had a colostomy bag for 14 years and was now in receipt of a PIP on top of his other benefits: "I get about £800 a month altogether; I don't really need to do the shops". He was, in effect, describing a *de facto* retirement from what had been almost a lifetime of his particular form of 'employment' (in fact, he had only ever worked legitimately for six months, sweeping up in a supermarket).

Paul, unlike Mack, gave up shoplifting many years ago. He told me that he had always done 'anything' to make money, and always on the wrong side of the law. He had done too many spells in prison; as he commented, with some pathos, he'd been caught too many times: "every time I walked into a shop, it was like I had a THIEF sign on my head". Paul has been 'on the sick' for the past 20 years. Some of that time has been spent in prison (see below) but otherwise he has lived alone, drinking heavily and taking a cocktail of drugs. In the research interview, I asked him how he could afford so much alcohol (and other things), the detail of which is later on:

---

47 This is a classic criminological theory relating to 'blocked opportunity structures' – see Cloward and Ohlin (1960). This particular group of the Boys were immersed in a criminal subculture.

Well I've been fiddling. That helps me through. Yeah, I can always get work, a few days here and there, fiddling, or whatever – look at me, whispering! – I suppose it's because, usually, I try not to let people know, because you do get people who don't like it if you're working and they might grass you up and then I'd get stopped claiming. On the buildings, labouring. I'm just a donkey. I'm not very well educated, so you couldn't give me instructions to cut something to length, but if somebody else marks it out, I can cut it.... I just do what they ask me...

Paul said he was taken on for different reasons. Sometimes people wanted some 'hard graft', but equally they sometimes just wanted some company. Either way, Paul was ready to be there, if asked; he'd pick up about £30 a day.

I reminded Paul that, in my role, in the mid-1970s, as a 'social and life skills training' instructor for a Job Creation Programme in Milltown, which had involved quite a number of the Boys, I had conducted a mock interview with him shortly after he officially left school. During the interview, he claimed to have experience of painting and decorating. When I asked how he had acquired it, he said calmly and factually "on the fiddle with the old man". This is what he had been doing, from time to time, for the previous two years (instead of going to school). I gently suggested that he needed to find a different way of explaining his 'work experience'[48]! Sadly, Paul has hardly ever worked legitimately since. Equally sadly, he bemoaned his lack of education and the fact that he had spent the whole of his life 'on the fiddle':

I probably haven't changed much since. I was never much good on the education. I always got stuck with words. I suppose if I could turn back the clock I would have done more of the education instead of sniffing glue!

Having been diagnosed with cancer, Ted was already in receipt of disability allowances totalling some £500 a month and a PIP of £140 a week. In early 2020,

---

48 My Wednesday afternoon job was to teach 'social and life skills' (SLS) to young people on the JCP, in order to prepare them for the world of work. There was no 'curriculum' beyond the Manpower Services Commission's *Instructional Guide to Social and Life Skills Training*. I had to make it up as I went along. With hindsight, I probably learned more about the Boys' 'world of work' than I prepared them for it. However, I discovered that many of the Boys were essentially illiterate and innumerate. They had no need to read or write (on the rare occasions they needed to, their mothers or sisters did it for them), and their arithmetic ability was sufficiently adept for them to work out a three-dart finish in a game of darts down the pub, but most struggled to divide 21 by 3. After one session where I covered basic numeracy, one of the Boys – not featured in my books, and not known for buying others a drink – was spotted buying *two* pints in *The Wayfarer* one evening after the SLS session that afternoon. As he put the extra pint down next to me (and it was *my* drink, a 'brown top' – half a bitter topped with brown ale), he whispered in my ear: "That's for you, How, and if you ever try to teach me sums again, I'll kill you". It might not have been a completely idle threat. Not long afterwards, he was sentenced to 15 years in prison for malicious wounding. Perhaps fortunately for me, he did not attend a 'social and life skills' session ever again.

he started to invest £40 a week in a credit union, to be sure of being able to finance a decent funeral. Ted observed that he might as well because he "didn't really need the money".

On the other side of 'earning' money through legitimate income there was also gambling, though some of the Boys struggled with new developments and the demise of the classical 'bookies'. There was, however, usually one amongst them who had won quite a lot, on the horses or the football, wins that were certainly counted in the hundreds and sometimes thousands of pounds. They talked about 'modern day' gambling, where you could place a bet on just about anything, in almost any way or combination you wanted, and followed this with the wonderful rejoinder that to win something decent "you still need to have a bit of luck". When I said I had never set foot in a betting shop, they were incredulous, promising to take me to one. They said it wasn't like the old days – paper, men, smoking and "the little shit pens that everybody used to nick". These days, they were more like an amusement arcade, with one-armed bandits, slot machines, coffee and even 'free money'. They waxed lyrical that if you signed up with on-line betting companies, you often got a free tenner: one of the Boys qualified his delight about this, "well it's not really free, 'cos you've got to spend it on a bet". They were not troubled by the thought that this was an incentive to hook you into playing with that company; after all, they said, they'd been gambling all their lives. They were not keen, however, on the technology of gambling, any more than they were keen on technology *per se*. Some of the Boys, in 2020, were still struggling with sending text messages on their mobile phones.

Few of these Boys held driving licences, yet all drove regularly and had access to a vehicle, the 'company car', as one quipped. Some taxed and insured their own vehicles (in other people's names), while others got friends and neighbours to do so. With the increased use of electronic surveillance of vehicles, they noted that there was little risk of getting 'pulled' so long as they were driving carefully, if tax and insurance were up to date. If checked, that would be legal; "nobody really cares who is driving"!

Those who had spent most of their lives operating on the wrong side of the law nevertheless drew attention to the fact that, on (rare) occasions, they had endeavoured to "be legit and go straight". Ted took umbrage when I alleged that he had never worked legitimately since a heavy industrial job when he was a teenager. He pointed out that he had once had a stall, selling cards, in a local market and, for a time, had worked for the council as a 'site supervisor' (in fact, as a security man). Neither job had lasted long; they simply did not provide much income. More recently, he did some roofing work for a couple of months but said it had nearly killed him. He'd also even done some volunteering work, ironically tidying up the garden at a nearby drug rehabilitation centre [!!]; his reasoning was that it had "helped to keep the social off my back".

Long ago, Danny had worked with his uncle on removals, but that didn't last long either. Danny also did a spell in conservation work, which provides him with a strong narrative about a legitimate working life, even though he didn't do it for long (but he now tells the respectable parents of his daughter's boyfriend that he is a retired tree surgeon). Much more recently, at the age of 57 and on a tag as a result of a conviction for shoplifting, he had worked with and for his younger brother, doing the 'mixing and cleaning' work that is needed when plastering:

> Working with Michael was hard work but I got used to it, quite enjoying it, as a plasterer's labourer – doing all the odd mixing and cleaning jobs required. I was earning £360 a week and I paid £60 in tax, so the tax office should be having a party to celebrate the first tax I've paid for over 30 years!

After only a few weeks, however, Danny had an argument with his brother and walked out. Despite his expressed intentions to stick at it – particularly as his nephew's three-year prison sentence for possession of cocaine had provided a sharp reminder of what might be in store for him should he have a further conviction for shoplifting (see below) – Danny has returned to his established modus operandi. Not that he sees it as offending; it is just a way of making a living, responding to market demand through the timely supply of requested items, rather as Tony also does, though on quite a different scale and on the other side of the law.

6

FAMILY AND RELATIONSHIPS

The Boys have continued to father children! Most are now grandfathers but some of those are now also older fathers of relatively young children. Danny, Ted, Matt and Vic (four of those, according to *The Milltown Boys Revisited* p.7, at the most pronounced end of deviance, social exclusion and marginality, both in 1975 and 2000) all have children who were born in the twenty-first century.

In 2000, the Boys in my study had 60 children between the 30 of them, though seven had no children (one, Pete, was gay; his first partner had no children, his second partner was bi-sexual and had two children by an earlier marriage). By 2020, they had fathered five more children, ranging in age from 16 to 10.

Matt, as ever, ended up in another tangle of relationships – he already had four children, by two different women, who were just two years apart (two are now 40, one 39 and one 38) – after release from a prison sentence in 2005. He met a 21-year-old girl, 24 years his junior ("I thought she was older and she thought I was younger"). Matt talked about relationships in terms of wearing handcuffs, and that particular one had ended before he discovered Marilyn was pregnant. His next relationship came to an abrupt halt when Sharlene learned that Matt was about to be the father of a child by another woman, born in 2009. Matt says he has a harmonious relationship with Marilyn (I interviewed him online when he was in her house), though he served a short custodial sentence for breaching a restraining order she had once taken out on him! His third – and by far the longest – relationship had not produced any children; his partner already had four children and Matt talks about them as his own – hence his claim to having 14 grandkids, even if 'only' 5 of them are through his own children.

Danny, who had married young but then divorced, has now been with his current partner Nathalie for 29 years, though they have never married ("she doesn't like wedding cake"). They had a second daughter, some 13 years after the birth of

TABLE 6.1 Relationships and children (developed from *The Milltown Boys Revisited*, p.124)

	Relationships and children						*Children at 2000 and since*	*Grandchildren*
	1st	2nd	3rd	4th	5th	6th		
Ted	1	2	2	2	0	0	5 + 2	15
Danny	0	2					1 + 1	1
Vic	1	3	1				4 + 1	2
Matt	2	2	0	1	0		4 + 1	5 + 9

the first. Vic separated from his partner and, for a while, formed another relationship, which produced a son but then unravelled, with consequences for both his working situation (see Chapter 6) and his living circumstances (see Chapter 10). Though he has always tried to have regular contact with this boy (now aged 13), he maintained that the system conspires heavily against fathers, rarely believing his side of the story:

> I had a bit of a breakdown. The relationship I was in, when I had the three kids, that broke down. We just weren't getting on. Then my mum and my grandmother died, within a month of each other. I wasn't coping tidy at all. But then I met this other woman, the mother of my boy. Then that went pear-shaped. She accused me of domestic abuse, which was unfounded. The problem was because we'd got a young son and we was arguing all the time, I'd gone to social services to ask for some help, but when they called the meeting, I was supposed to have been the bad person. I wasn't allowed to explain. I was trying to stand up for myself because I was being bullied. So I joined this group for men in abusive relationships. I just couldn't cope. I went to the NSPCC and to the Children's Society. I offered to go on a course, voluntarily. I completed the course. I interacted. I challenged other fathers to talk more about what was going on in their lives, just to tell the truth. I was open and honest. Things went back and forth, but eventually I lost everything. I lost my house, I lost my job, I lost access to my son. I'd had my son, on my own, for a while, because there was a time when she didn't want him. I tried to tell social services, but nobody wanted to know my side of the story. It was all about his mum, how she was the victim. No, I was the victim; where men are concerned in these situations, they don't want to know. You know, Howard, I was treated like shit, by social services, by CAFCASS. The first thing the guy from CAFCASS [the Children and Family Court Advisory and Support Service] said to me was did you know that nine out of ten black men leave their children. I said I never left my son, I just left his mother. When I went to the civil court, even the judge said he could see I was trying to do the right thing, but she still wouldn't let me see him, and now I can't

because I ended up having trouble with Robert's mum's boyfriend. My boy was a bit upset one day and I took it out on the boyfriend. I filled him in. I was honest with the police about it. I went to court. I pleaded guilty. I got fined and they put me on a Relationship course and I was still challenging that they don't do nothing for men; it's all about the women. I ended up on my own. It was after that that I went off sailing round the world.

Ted had a relatively short spell in prison in 2003 – he wrote to me at the university, telling me proudly that he had done GCSE English and a health and safety course – only to discover, on release, that his partner had been 'playing around', so he "got rid of her and found another woman". This relationship produced two boys, aged 14 and 11 in 2020, but it did not last. Ted moved on to his fifth 'serious' relationship in 2012, certainly serious enough to get married to Lucy, in Thailand in 2015. Soon afterwards, however, they split up and Ted has since shared his life with Althea, who lives just up the road and who has, he proclaims, "made me a better person". She sometimes stays with him; he sometimes stays with her. "Depends how I feel", Ted commented, "that way, she doesn't get in the way". Nonetheless, with his cancer diagnosis and the Covid-19 crisis, which consigns him to a 'vulnerable' group (though he adamantly resists the label!), it is either Althea or his youngest daughter, Hayley, who does his shopping while he remains in self-isolation. In the research interview, Ted recurrently referred to Althea as his 'rock'.

Keeping up with his grandchildren seemingly poses no problem for Ted. Even if he may not get on with all of their grandmothers, he said, they are all 'one big happy family', all getting on *with each other*. And not one of them would be here were it not for him, he says forcefully, stating the blindingly obvious! They all come over at Christmas (photos of these impressive family gatherings are always posted on Facebook) and although some are already grown up while others are babies he has a simple approach to presents in order to avoid arguments and keep things simple: "a hundred pounds each family, whatever the number of kids".

Most of the Boys in *The Milltown Boys Revisited* have remained with their part-ners from those days. Suzanne, Tommy's wife, now suffers from memory loss as a result of an embolic stroke; she also has regular fits. At a party to celebrate Kelvin's wife Julie's 60th birthday, I broke a golden rule by venturing over to say hello to the 'women' and very intentionally sat next to Suzanne. She had no idea who I was, though after some cajoling and reminding by some of the others she commented vaguely 'from up the Rec'. I was not sure whether this was a statement of recog-nition or a question. I could not tell whether or not she remembered me. One of their children, Vanessa, had connected with me on Facebook, and I had written to ask after her parents:

Hi Howard yes I do remember you of course dad still has his book. And yes all good here mum and dad are ok, mum does get confused especially remembering people but that's due to her embolism she does really well considering. I shall pass on your message to them both, so how are you? Hope you are well?

Later I heard that Tommy and Suzanne's son, Raymond, is the father of triplets, so while Tommy cares for his wife (having retired to do so), she looks after the 'handful' who are her five years old grandchildren.

Long after my conversation with Vanessa in her parents' garden when she was 14, about the cultural tensions resulting from coming from Milltown but mixing with the children of doctors and lawyers at school, I learned that she had dropped out of the elite private school, to which she had gained a scholarship, before taking any exams. By chance, I had paid a visit to the social club they frequented around the time it happened. Suzanne told me about Vanessa and then immediately asked me to go to see Tommy, who was playing skittles. I went through the skittle alley where a match was in full swing. But Tommy took me to one side. He was a mixture of tears and fury – that Vanessa was throwing up such an opportunity. He said how helpless they felt but there seemed little they could do about it.

Danny's daughter, Cathy, got a scholarship from the same school. She, too, dropped out before she was 16, withdrawn by Danny before he anticipated she would be expelled:

> Cathy could've been anything. She could have been what she wanted to be. The headmistress told us that. She was so bright,[49] intelligent, patient, clever. But she met this girl – I know it's not nice to blame somebody else – but this girl was always on the piss, and Cathy climbed on the wagon with her. And at the school, this girl called her names, and she retaliated, so I had to take her out, so she didn't have on her record that she'd been expelled from a school like that. And she started running away from home and then she moved away and she worked in restaurants and other things, and then she had Alfie. She was on her own so I got her to move back down here, and now Alfie lives with us a lot.... So it's like I was as a kid, cos I spent more time over here, in Milltown, with my grandparents than I did over Fairfield with my mum and dad.

Danny's younger daughter has at least reached her mock GCSEs, worked hard for them, and is planning to stay on at school to do 'A' levels alongside her particular crowd of friends.[50]

---

49 Fathers invariably say this, particularly about their daughters. However, when I was a board member of the Youth Justice Board, I chaired meetings of magistrates. By chance in a casual conversation with one J.P., it transpired she taught in one of Milltown's junior schools. When I remarked that such work must be quite challenging, she retorted that there were 'unexpected rewards', highlighting the occasional exceptionally bright pupil – and, by way of example, she mentioned Danny's daughter by name! I did not reveal my connection.

50 Danny places a lot of store by the influence of friendship groups, maintaining that Cathy got in with the wrong crowd, while Ophelia is in with a good crowd. When I asked him about himself as a teenager, he paused and simply said "**I** was the wrong crowd"!

It was at the funeral of the wife of one of the Boys who was not featured explicitly in my last study that Spaceman renewed contact with Kate, who had been the only girl to actively 'hang out' with the Boys in their younger days. When Spaceman came to talk to my students in November 2019, Kate gave him a lift to the university and joined the session, contributing her own experience and perceptions of the Boys; I had not seen her for almost exactly 40 years (not since early December 1979)! We remained in touch; Kate celebrated her own 60th birthday in June 2020. The party she had planned was, however, cancelled because of the Covid-19 situation. Kate knew I was writing the book and when she sent a message to let me know that her party was not going ahead, asked "How's the book coming along at least you have more time to do it at the moment?" In her teenage years, she had first met the Boys in a noisy bar and when one of them had asked what she did, she had said, jokingly, that she was a 'psychic'. He had thought she said 'psycho', and the name stuck. After she lost touch with the Boys, she did a number of things, ranging from being a 'hand model' to working on child development! Now, when I said that much of the book had been written (early June 2020), she revealed that one of her sons had just graduated in medicine:

> Wow my son finished his dissertation on Sunday, who would have thought all those years ago living in Milltown I would actually give birth to a doctor lol. He did physiology (after his mum phyco lol) he did it at Exeter he had a choice between there and ucl. Life is strange I left school without an 'O' level. I think I did well considering my upbringing. I'm a strong believer in putting the past behind you and striving for what you want in life, it's out there and determination is the key.

Someone like Gary would certainly agree, even though he separated from his wife Amelia some years ago. They have, however, remained on good terms and in regular contact. Gary is very forthright for the reasons for the breakdown of their relationship:

> I was in the way. I'd been working away and she did everything for the kids and then I'd come home and, more and more, I could tell that I was getting on her nerves. I still love her to bits. I've spoken to her twice this week. She's done so much for me. Her father's a Milltown boy but she grew up elsewhere, although they did move back here. I met her when I was 19. She helped me so much with my English. I owe her a lot. It was my choice to split up. It wasn't just the work. Adrian was also misbehaving all the time and it all got too much. I could see the strain on Amelia and I decided it would be better if I left.

In my research interview with Gary, I had little choice but to broach the emotive and sensitive topic of Adrian's suicide. Adrian took his own life in 2018; he was 24. Gary had said in the past that he had often expected to find Adrian at the end of a rope, knowing about his addictions, mood swings and lack of sense of purpose in the world. Adrian had taken an overdose, with drugs bought on the dark web. That night Gary had left his mobile phone in his van and in the morning discovered four missed calls from Adrian; when Spaceman called to tell me the tragic news, he commented "God know how that must be affecting him".

Only about a year before Adrian's suicide, Gary, Spaceman and I had had a pub meal together. Gary had, once again, expressed concern about his son, particularly his drinking. Gary, as we know, has always been a phenomenally hard-working individual, a trait he claims he inherited from his father. He deplored Adrian's 'lay-about' lifestyle, loved him dearly and was desperate to know what he might do to help. During the meal, quite by chance, Adrian called his father; the two of them had an amiable exchange and afterwards Gary commended his 'boy' as basically a decent kid who couldn't find any direction in his life. There was some suggestion he might be gay. He shared a flat with another young man. But he had never talked about it, and Gary really didn't want to ask. But Gary's words in the pub were a powerful, and soon afterwards poignant, analysis. And in fact, shortly before Adrian died, Gary *had* asked him if he was gay; Adrian had retorted that it was none of his business.

Spaceman notified me by text about the funeral. No black, at Adrian's request, he said: "his favourite colour was pink". Then even later on the same day, he sent me another text:

> Spoke with Gary I am going out with him tomorrow he wants me to do a painting of Adrian. He seems ok but I think he is still in shock. We spoke for about 30 minutes. So I went out and bought a pink Ralph Lauren shirt for the funeral – Adrian would love it. He was chuffed when I told him that you said, "call me – if there's anything I can do" he understood fully! He says hello but you will probably hear from him anyway. x

Adrian had a humanist service to celebrate his life. He had prepared the script, including the request that all men attending should wear something pink. Everybody did. Sixteen of the 30 Boys I had interviewed in 2000 were there, in one or another of pink socks, shirts, ties and scarves. Danny would've come had he been informed, but he said later that he hadn't known about it. Glenn Webbe, the Welsh international rugby player (see above), a lifelong friend of Gary's, was there. So, to my surprise, was one of my PhD students who, unknown to me, was an old school friend of Amelia's.

Though nothing explicit was said about him being gay, much was said about Adrian's sensitive nature, his love of reading, his interest in and later use of cosmetics and make-up, his care for animals and his consideration for others. His choice of songs and poems was also very telling, in relation to the mental health problems he had clearly experienced; donations were requested for 'Heads Together', the mental health charity formed by the Duke and Duchess of Cambridge and Prince Harry. It was a very moving moment. It was also the moment when, following a sequence of remarks by many of the Boys, it became clear to me that I should try to write another book.

In reflecting on Adrian's passing, when I broached the subject during the research interview, Gary said that he didn't mind talking about it:

> I'm through that, H. Of course, I still think about him every day. Of course I do. But you've got to move on.
>
> I just think Adrian lost his way. He didn't care anymore. He was a clever kid but he never wanted to work. He thought hard work was only for idiots and donkeys. He always had the right answers to everything but he never kept his word. I think he was a bit like Marty. He had mental illness. He was away with the fairies. I could never put my finger on it, but that's what I think now.
>
> He left school at 16. He could have done better, in my view. But he'd started running with a bad crew and had got into a lot of trouble with the law. The police were often round the house.
>
> Amelia knew he was different. I'm pretty sure of that. Whereas perhaps I denied it and now we'll never know. I took him to the football and I took him quad biking. I hoped he would turn the corner but he never did. I remember I took him to work with me. He was about 18. It was down in Maidstone. I thought it might help but after three days he'd had a gut's full and went home. He just got on a train and went home. In that sort of way he was confident. Nothing phased him.
>
> Oh, it was awful times. He was just so ill. He did see a shrink but they said there was nothing wrong.
>
> I know he was using a lot of drugs. He got them off the dark web. He was always experimenting. He mixed with a lot of naughty boys; for some reason, he identified with them. I don't know what went wrong. I'll never know.

Gary spends a lot of time, these days, with his three grandchildren, taking them to Dominos for a pizza and trying to understand their use of technology. His daughter, Simone, had gone to university but left to work for his sister, who has her own business providing social care. Simone had her first child at 19 and two more at 22 and 25. All, Gary noted proudly, were planned! At 60, and despite the sadness over Adrian, Gary remains full of vitality – "I might occasionally need a grandad nap, but I've still got bags of energy and I'm a loving grandfather".

The children of the Boys have had very mixed trajectories, including the extent of contact with their fathers. When I discovered that one of Ted's sons was a 'friend' on Facebook of one of my former students, now a PhD student looking at the positive dimensions of male manual labour, I wrote to the latter to find out how they knew each other:

> Yeah, I've known him [Robbie, now 35] for years; he's a good guy. I used to play rugby against him, and he now coaches C. youth and I coach S. (local rivalry). I'm good thanks. Hope you are too.

Tony's two daughters, Katy and Hannah (now mothers with two girls and one boy, respectively) both work for his company. Katy's husband is the European manager of an I.T. company; Hannah's partner, who also works for the company, is the son of Tony's business partner. Katy had joined an architect's office on leaving school and done various qualifications on the job before joining Tony's company a couple of years ago. Hannah, now 33, studied Fashion and Design at university, but had never applied it in working life. She joined the company when Tony became a partner. Tony observed that she had only just "scraped through" having spent three years "just having a great time" and suggesting that her qualities really lay in "engaging with people, so she is very customer facing… she must take after me!". Yet, despite their social mobility and a very different lifestyle, some solid Milltown traditions remain: they both live close to their parents and, beyond work, see them most days.

Jamie's two children are much the same. They, too, don't live so far away from their parents. Both attended a Russell Group university and have gone on to pursue professional careers, Jack (now 31) in digital marketing and Roisin (now 29) in occupational therapy. Yet, once again, the cultural legacy of Milltown played its part in assisting their career trajectories, certainly for Jack, if only oiling the wheels of opportunity. As Jamie recounts:

> Well they both lived at home while they were studying, so I suppose they missed out on not going away to somewhere like Glasgow. They were spoilt, I suppose. Me and the wife looked after them. We got them jobs and so they left with no debts. They were both lifeguards at the leisure centre….
>
> And then it was out into the big, wide world and I was talking to a mate in the skittles team… well, all our sons at one time or another were 'sticker-uppers' for the skittles team.[51] So I happened to be talking to one of the team, who'd once been a sticker-upper himself, and he said he was in I.T. And I told him my son had just graduated in I.T. and he said, 'as it happens we're looking for someone and we'll take on graduates', so Jack met him, got the job, and he was happy as Larry. And I said thank you very much to the fella who'd taken him on, for doing me a favour, like… you know, the old saying, it's who you know. He stopped me in my tracks and said, 'Jamie, he got the job on merit, it was nothing to do with you'. And I smiled and offered to buy him a drink, but he went on, praising Jack up to the hilt for the way he'd performed in his interview. Yeah, he said all this nice stuff about Jack and I said to him, 'do me a favour if you will – don't tell him that, because as far as Jack knows, I got him the job!'

51 Jamie asked me 'Have you played skittles?' Before I could answer, he said that

> a sticker-upper is the kid who sticks them up, puts up the nine wooden skittles (it's not like ten pin) … And in all the years we've been playing, our kids have 'stuck-up' for us. It's good money. Now it's about twelve quid, for two and a half hours, perhaps even a bit more. Maybe even fifteen quid. That's all right for a little ten-year old kid, isn't it?

Jamie grinned. All the jobs *he'd* ever had were always acquired through word of mouth and he hadn't really realised the world had changed. Gordon's daughters had also gone to university, with the younger one, Melissa, spending a semester at Melbourne Business School. The more successful of the Boys (in terms of their relationships) have conferred even brighter futures on many of their children, or at least consolidated different possibilities for them. Kelvin's three children, for example, are a self-employed delivery driver (with three young children), a seller of health and fitness products (with one child, who lives with Kelvin and his wife) and a store manager for Virgin Media (engaged to be married). As he proudly told me their occupational stories, he said he couldn't complain: "they're all doing well and are in good health, touch wood".

The life course for many of the other children has been rather more hit and miss. Mack's son, Stuart, for example, had become the world junior pool champion as a teenager, and subsequently toured many parts of the world and featured in a number of YouTube videos. At the age of 12, Stuart was already excelling on the pool table, as reported in *The Milltown Boys Revisited* (p.150):

> Not a lot of money is yet to be made from these talents, and the Boys *in The Fountain* have a whip-round to send Stuart and Mack off to tournaments and exhibitions, but Mack considers this to be the 'career' route Stuart should be taking – and he is already a very competent 'hustler' on the pool table in the pub!

Success has been more elusive in recent years and Stuart set up his own plastering and roofing company (essentially as a sole trader), though he still plays sponsored exhibition matches where he receives about 20% of the takings. Now 32, Stuart has moved back to Milltown and lives just down the road from Mack. He has three daughters (aged 15, 10 and 6), by three different mothers, two of whom live in Milltown, while the other does not live far away. Mack sees all his grandchildren regularly. His own daughter, Andrea, does not have children and works in the canteen at a nearby hospital.

Mark's son, Colin, is a panel beater, with two children aged 11 and 8. His daughter, Eirlys, is a dinner lady (as his sister had been). Mark noted proudly that "all the women in our family work in schools" (though none as teachers). Eirlys (now aged 35) has three children by two different fathers. One of the older two, who is already 16, lives with his father; the other two, a girl of 11 and a boy of 8, live with her. Mark says he sees them all, from time to time.

Some relationships have also continued to blow hot and cold. Mack was once on the verge of splitting up with his wife when she gave him an ultimatum about his excessive drug use (mainly amphetamines) but he curtailed his habit and they have remained together ever since. Trevor had also, long ago, separated from and then reunited with his wife, but they are now divorced. Trevor has remarried and has a 20-year-old stepdaughter and five grandchildren between the ages of 7 and 20.

Ted has had three further 'serious' relationships since 2000, the first producing two more children, the second leading to marriage and the third romantic-
ally presented – on Facebook – on Valentine's Day 2020, as 'best girlfriend ever'.
A week later, he was visited by his eldest son and one of Andy's six children (by
three different women), aged 10, Ted's daughter by his third relationship and her
daughter, aged 8; Ted was quick to tell me that:

> Although my children have a lot of different mothers, the kids and the
> grandkids all get on as one big family, there's no 'step' or 'half' or any of that,
> they're just a big family, cursing and blinding each other all the time!

With 7 children by 4 different women, and 15 grandchildren, all of whom he sees
regularly, he had a point.

It is worth dwelling on Ted for a little longer. He came from a very large family: ten
boys and three girls. His parents died at about the same time when Ted, second from
youngest, was 12. In his own words, he became an 'uncontrollable kid'. His eldest
sister, at 19 already a mother, tried to look after the four youngest siblings, but –
rather predictably – struggled. Ted was surrounded by offending and had already
been socialised into shoplifting and other forms of petty crime. He was taken into
care and sent to a children's home a long way from 'home'. His eldest sister Rhian
married a notorious (legendary) rogue from a large English city, attached to a network of criminals "who were not to be messed with". All the 'boys' in the family,
bar one, were enmeshed in criminality and the 'girls' were too, if only by association. Ted's little sister died very young – like their mother, in her 30s – of throat
cancer; many of his brothers were also dead before they were 50. His slightly older
brother then turned a corner and became something of a community activist in
Milltown, organising fund-raising discos and social walks through the nearby woods,
and campaigning about escalating energy bills. One of his older sisters, married to
a Londoner (known to all as 'Cockney Pete'), celebrated her 40th wedding anniversary in 2020. Even more striking was that Rhian, after her daughter-in-law
was diagnosed with breast cancer and losing three of her four sons in the space of
12 years,[52] set about raising money for a nearby cancer hospital. For that fund-raising
endeavour, she was awarded a British Citizen Award in 2018, which she received at
the Palace of Westminster. The accolade was widely reported in the local media and
Ted's older brother posted a tribute on Facebook:

[edited for confidentiality]

I have wonderful news for Milltown and my family.

When you lose four of your brothers and a sister, mother and father at an
early age, it is easy to just say "enough is enough" and just give up.

---

52 The youngest died in 2005, aged 25, in a car crash. Another, who suffered from epilepsy, died, aged
41, of a seizure, in 2016. The third, aged 38, had an unexpected stroke six months later, in 2017.

That is what has happened to me and my sisters.

So just imagine when that happens then you lose 3 sons, 2 in the last 12 months.

That takes it to a much higher level.

Despite all this happening to my sister Rhian, one disaster after another and not knowing when it is going to cease, she could have been forgiven if she had forgotten that she has grandchildren to support, and who could blame her?

She could also be forgiven for not caring about people who are ill.

But today, I can proudly announce to my family and Milltown that Rhian Hodges nee Nash has been awarded in the New Year's Honours list and will receive the BCA (British Citizens' Award) medal on 25 January.

The medal is awarded for services to the community in the category of volunteering and giving Rhian and some of her family and friends have been working rigorously, day in, day out, raising funds for the Breast Cancer Unit and to date has raised £60,000.

Not many people that were nominated made the final cut but their committee decided what Rhian had achieved was significant and inspirational, especially under the extraordinary circumstances.

I have to say that I totally agree their decision and am so proud of this lady. She really is an inspiration to us all.

She has shown that no matter who you are, where you are from or what life can chuck at you, there is always room for courage, love and even just a bit of consideration for others who may need some help.

Our family and a few friends will be travelling to Westminster Palace on January 25 for Rhian to accept the award.

Well done girl, not bad for a Woolworth counter girl.

Your boys, Mam and Dad, brothers and sisters would be so proud of you too.

Enjoy your success and sail on. Keep showing us how to brush off any small adversity and teach us how we can turn around negative events into a powerful force for good.

May I also take this opportunity to thank all her supporters, family and friends for the amazing help, unselfishly and consistently given to my sister especially in the darker moments. I know she feels the same.

At the time of writing [2020], Rhian had raised £134,000 for her cause. The family name has come to be seen in a different light.

Ted's view was that his own family was paramount. Notwithstanding the breakups with their mothers, he had maintained or renewed positive contact with all of his seven children, noting proudly that "no matter what, I've supported my kids, and now my grandkids, whether they are right or wrong". He waxed lyrical about having bought Robbie his first car, made sure that others had been properly kitted out for school and taken most of the boys to many a rugby game.

Far from the complex 'reconstituted' families that prevail in the lives of Ted, Vic and Matt, some of the other Boys have remained with their childhood sweethearts or partners from early adulthood. Jamie met Phoebe when they were teenagers and "although we had some time apart at the start, we've always been together". Kelvin and Julie have been together throughout their adult lives ("37 years, quite an achievement.... So haven't done too badly"), as have Tony and Angie who, in July 2020, celebrated 35 years of marriage.

Gary may have parted from his wife, but he still speaks to her most days. Danny may have had a short marriage and divorce in his early 20s, but he has been with his current partner ever since, though they have never married. They have 2 children who are, as already noted, 13 years apart, and a 5-year-old grandson Alfie, on whom Danny dotes and with whom he spends a great deal of time.

Paul has four children, three boys by one relationship and a daughter by another. During the research interview, he reminded me three times, almost proudly, that his youngest son and his daughter are just four *months* apart. Those almost parallel births destroyed Paul's relationships with both mothers and poisoned his relationships with most of his children. He was 'with' the mother of his daughter, after a fashion, for six years but then she left. She had lived next door to his sister who called him one day to say that the neighbour's house was empty:

> She'd gone, took my 5-year old daughter with her, and I've never seen her since. I went to Family Mediation to try to find her, but nothing happened. So I gave up.

He still sees his oldest son "quite often", and his middle son "sometimes, when he wants to use my flat to shag some girl", though the latter otherwise has little to do with him. His youngest son, now 25, is gay and doesn't speak to him at all. Perhaps unaware of the direct implications of his words, Paul commented,

> They hate my guts. I bite my tongue. Yeah, it's sad but you've still got to try to have a laugh. I've made my bed, so I've got to lie on it.

Within seconds of starting the research interview, when I opened my questions asking whether or not Paul lived on his own, he forthrightly confirmed that he hadn't been with a woman since I last interviewed him. Perhaps he'd had sex twice, he said, in 20 years. Later in the interview, he observed poignantly,

> I've probably forgotten how to date a woman. I'd like to, but it don't happen. I wouldn't know how. Everybody says I've got a lovely personality. I could talk to one. I can have a laugh and a joke with a woman. I can fancy them, but I don't think I'd know how to chat one up. Maybe I never did, not even

the ones I had kids with. Maybe I just fucked them anyway and that just produced the kids!

His oldest son has three children, a boy and two girls. The oldest is 17, the girls are 10 and 6. His middle son has a son of six. Paul doesn't see them a lot, but makes sure he does so on their birthdays:

> I know all their birthdays. I always sort them out, you know, their birthdays, and at Christmas. I might not have been a very good father, but I've tried to be a better grandparent. I try harder now.

I asked him how he had felt when his youngest boy had come out as gay. After all, in homophobic Milltown of the 1970s, the only gay man known to the Boys was Pete who, soon after coming out as gay, had 'escaped' to London and never returned. Paul made some interesting remarks:

> Yeah, my youngest boy is gay. Because of that, I thought he might have some sympathy for me, but he's done nothing for me. That's the one who don't talk to me. I've tried over the years with him, but nothing happens.
>
> I had a feeling about it before he come out with it. I didn't say anything to his mother but I just felt it, like that. He didn't come out with it until he was about 16 or 17. It was my middle boy who told me. He said 'I've got something to tell you' and he said, 'Lewis is bi-sexual'. And I said I already knew that. I'd been looking at him since he was about 10 and was thinking that he was like that. I'm not saying it's not right, being like that. Some people think we don't talk because he's gay and I don't like it, but it's not that at all. He don't wanna talk to me because of what I done. I'm not saying that what he's like is right or wrong. I don't care. People have got to be what they wanna be. There's a lot more people gay now than when I was growing up. Or they're more open about it. I've read that every family's got someone who's gay, either their own family or a relative, like a cousin. Something's happening. It's more open, isn't it? The only one we knew was Pete. If I'd wanted to be gay in them days, I would've been battered, by my parents and in the street. It just wasn't acceptable.

Pete and Barry, incidentally, have now been together for well over 30 years.

For Danny, bringing up children and grandchildren "was the best thing that ever happened to me":

> Until I was 32 I was nothing, I thought I was nothing, 'cos I didn't have any kids. And when I did, it changed me, I started behaving myself. I don't class what I do now as getting into trouble [see below], whereas before I was always getting into trouble, big trouble, through fighting and all those other things. I'd done a lot of time, but I didn't think so much about it. It was just

what you did. But now I had to start thinking of other people. I used to go for things – burglaries, robberies. You know, I just didn't care what the consequences were. Either I got away with it or I didn't. But when the kids come along, I thought I don't want to be away for a long time… and the helicopter. That put a stop to the robberies, but it was mainly the kids that calmed me down. I don't think I would've stopped if I'd never had children.

And now I've got Alfie, and I spend so much time with him, over the woods. We went camping the other day. I spent all my spare time with him.

Like some of the other Boys, as noted above, Danny has rarely worked legitimately, but sees himself fundamentally as a family man, whose offending behaviour is justified primarily in terms of providing for the kids.

7

CRIME

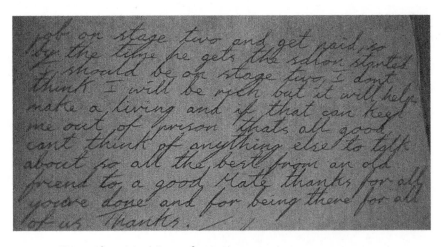

PHOTO 2 Extract from Matt's Letter from prison

Matt's plans to open a hairdressing salon – thought up, as noted above, in 2007 after doing a National Vocational Qualification (NVQ) in 'barbering' while serving an 18-month prison sentence for robbery – in the hope it might keep him out of prison never materialised. Instead, since I last interviewed him, Matt has been involved in an aborted attempt at international drug smuggling and has cleaned the chandeliers in the central London branch of Jimmy Choo! The first activity is too sensitive to report, though it ended with the fatal shooting of two of Matt's collaborators. [This was certainly *not* 'more Monty Python than Al Capone', as one of the Boys had depicted their offending behaviour in *The Milltown Boys Revisited* (pp.67–98)!] Matt made a hasty return, empty-handed, to the UK saying that if he was going to get done for anything, "at least I'd go to a British jail". Although he stood to make tens of thousands of pounds if everything came off, Matt concluded that "nothing has ever worked for me". Then his youngest son was conceived and Matt rejoined the cleaning firm he had been employed by in the past (see Chapter 6). There has been no more instrumental offending, though he has been convicted five times for assaulting the police and was sent to prison at the age of 57 for breaching a restraining order – in Matt's eyes, yet another episode of injustice, given that his son's mother had invited him to her house and then reported him for being there. In a similar vein, Vic had been fined £150 and made subject to a three-year restraining order for 'filling in' (beating up) his youngest son's mother's boyfriend. He was insistent that this was his only 'trouble' with the law since his much younger days:

> Howard, the only problem I've ever had since I had all my children has been with my son Robert's mum. I've never been in any trouble since my 20s. And I've never been convicted of any domestic abuse. There's been no charges against me. Every time I've been accused of it, they've taken me to the police station, spoken to me, and said to me you can go. There's no charges. I was the one who was the victim all the time. You know, there was one time, I went to watch my boy play rugby and the next I knew was the police were there wanting to speak to me because his mum had phoned them to say I had threatened to murder her. And I said to them that they had my record and knew exactly what I was about. I've got no convictions for beating women up. It's not my style. If I wanted to beat anybody up, I'd beat the boyfriends up.
>
> When I had a breakdown, I talked a lot to the community psychiatric team, and they had to tell the police that I'm not capable of that sort of thing. I'm not horrible. If I wanted to be, I could be, easily.
>
> She just don't want me around. She's got three other children by three different fathers and none of them have anything to do with their children. Whereas I do, and she tries to stop it. Although she once told Robert that she didn't want him anymore and he phoned me, so I went to get him from school and took him back the next day. Then when I went to pick him up that afternoon, she'd already taken him home. And she'd told social services I had taken him away, which I just wouldn't do, because I know every kid really wants to be with their mum.

Vic has always *looked* like a 'hard' man and he had been a wayward teenager, serving time in custody. [His eldest son does conform to the stereotype of the luxury car driving, black guy in dark glasses, dealing drugs; at the age of 25, he has already spent more than a decade in custody.] As Vic said in *The Milltown Boys Revisited* (p.224), as he ruminated that he was really quite a 'sensitive, considerate bloke' concealed within a 'big bloke with a loud voice': "People look at me and they think that's Vic, criminal record, hard case, he's a thief". He suggested that "you get known for being a thief and being a fighter and it stays with you". How right he was.

Shoplifting, like politics, is the art of the possible. Those of the Boys involved in this particular form of offending had, increasingly, to operate further and further away from home. They were too well known, by storekeepers, security officers, and the police – and easily recognised on CCTV. Further afield, and this came to be well over one hundred miles away, they were not. But their 'work' became quite a sophisticated operation, requiring initial reconnaissance, further exploration and experimentation. Sometimes, wearing the right gear to avoid technological identification, it was possible literally to 'sweep' a range of items into a bag and make a run for it, often lobbing the bag to a partner, making off down a side-street and then mingling with a crowd. Sometimes it was not. Yet these Boys invoked so many ruses, apologies and explanations that, despite this being their *daily* round, few have served any custodial sentences for many years. When I mentioned to one of them that the last time he had been inside had been almost 20 years ago, he sighed and told me not to tempt fate. It would be a breach of my confidentiality to the Boys to reveal more of the logistics of their shoplifting strategies, save to say that they have an armoury of them that militate against the chances of being caught red-handed. Few go back home with any stolen property, because they already have cash in hand, having exchanged their ill-gotten gains along the way. Bizarrely, everything has to be based on *trust* and it was not unknown for a recipient to call to say that a bag of items was the equivalent of £20 or £30 short because only a 3-pack rather than a 4-pack of something or other had been stolen. The Boys always rectified the 'error', knowing how dependent they are on their 'fences',[53] but only through supplementing the next supply: "we never do cash refunds", one of the Boys joked, in absolute seriousness. [It is worth noting that my research interviews with the Boys were conducted mainly during the Covid-19 lockdown, when most shops were closed and the police were also having considerable success in detecting illegal behaviour requiring the transfer of contraband through road checks of the relatively few drivers on the road. Both contexts meant that those Boys engaged in such activities had had to review their lifestyles. As Mack said, in his inimitable capacity to state the blindingly obvious: "you can't go out shoplifting if there aren't any shops open"! Danny, however, as we shall see below, had other ideas.]

In their younger days, the Boys were involved in a wide repertoire of offending behaviour, from armed robbery, credit card fraud, drug running and dealing, property and vehicle theft, shoplifting, illegal substance misuse and more besides. Today, those still involved in any criminality (and many have desisted completely, often many years ago) have generally narrowed down their criminal enterprise to dealing 'less harmful' drugs and shoplifting. They explain this in a number of ways, though

---

53 Carl Klockars, in his book *The Professional Fence* (Tavistock 1975), describes a 'fence' as a go-between for customers and thieves, the 'receiver' of stolen goods. Klockars' study provides a fascinating insight into being a 'fence', through a life-history analysis of the work of one man, 'Vincent Swaggi', whom he interviewed over 15 months. The book was described by Norman Denzin (1975), in a review for the *American Journal of Sociology*, as having restored 'sociological respectability to the life-history, ethnographic method'.

largely to minimise risk and reduce the prospects of doing more 'jail time'. Most are convinced that, in the relatively unlikely scenario of a conviction, their 'clean' record for some years should produce a non-custodial sentence. They are probably right.

Why do they carry on at all? First of all, even if the legitimate labour market would have them, the pay they would be likely to get is not, in their eyes, enough. One or two have tried a few days of quasi-legitimate employment. Danny had earned £360 a week (for a few weeks), working for his brother, significantly less than he routinely produced through his illegal activities. Notwithstanding the low pay, the work routines were too demanding and the work was sometimes described as 'too hard'. At least in the illegal labour market, they were 'self-employed' and their own boss: when they made money it was theirs, when they failed to make money, it was their own fault.

Danny had been almost compelled into working with his brother, both on account of fear about another conviction for shoplifting and being incapacitated from earning a living in that way as a result of a driving ban and being on a tag that restricted his movements (and options). This had caused at least a brief reflection on his lifestyle, particularly as his nephew had recently been sent to prison for three years for possession of cocaine. When Danny had visited, he was starkly reminded of what it was like to be banged up. Danny himself had been prosecuted for stealing £100.00 worth of goods from a well-known supermarket. Though he has nearly 100 criminal convictions, going back to the age of 14, when he was fined £5.00 for taking a vehicle without the owner's consent, he has rarely (in relative terms!) been caught for shoplifting, even though it is his 'daily work':

> Normally, as you know, How, I don't mess about. I just plead guilty and accept the fine. But I was up for something else which I never done, and they told me that if I was found guilty I could go to prison, so I'd better have legal representation. I hadn't been caught for over four years, and anyway I was found not guilty for the other offence, but they said that I was going to be up before [magistrate] who's known for being hard on 'persistent' offenders. And every one of my previous 20 convictions is for shoplifting! So, anyway, I got done for the one charge and he [magistrate] told me he'd still been thinking of sending me to prison. I got fined £600.00 and put on a 6pm to 7am curfew with a tag, so I can't leave the house in the evening and at night, or early in the morning. And I got banned from driving for six months.

'Early in the morning' is significant, as Danny drove long distances to commit his offences, to somewhere he was unlikely to be recognised and where he would probably not be on record; his 'working day' was something like 6 a.m. to midday and he would be back in Milltown by around 2 p.m., when – in the past – he would link up with other Boys in the pub. As he was telling me this story, he showed me the tag around his ankle and the box by the TV that sounds the alarm at the local police station if the perimeter is breached, though he spent more time complaining that the colour of the box did not match the colour scheme in his living room! The conviction, and the threat of prison once again, had at the time (2017) provided food for thought and had been a possible 'wake up time' moment (see *The Milltown Boys Revisited*, pp.230–233):

> Now I'm working, I've probably put all that behind me. You know, when I went to see my nephew, I was glad I've left all that behind. I've had over 25 good years of shoplifting. I can earn a bit less now. We sold the horses for a few hundred pounds because Ophelia [younger daughter] wasn't so interested. So I don't need so much and I can spend a bit more time with Alfie [his three-year old grandson]. The worst thing about losing my licence is I can't take him anywhere in the car.

But Danny had gone back to his old ways, even during the Covid-19 lockdown when there were new product lines that were worth lifting. Navigating the socially distanced queues outside supermarkets was a new challenge but he had risen to it: "I only does a couple of days a week now; I only does it for him [grandson]. I don't need the money. I never spend anything on myself".

Danny's reasoning is quite fascinating and palpably rational. In 20 years, he estimates he has been caught no more than 15 or 16 times – less than once a year. Until the most recent conviction, the only penalties imposed were financial, bar once, when he was required to do 60 hours of community service. Financial penalties simply demand a bit more effort 'at work', in order to pay the fine. Overall, Danny estimates he's had a total of around £10,000 in fines. He reckons his recent conviction led to a six-month tag only because he refused to reveal the name of the person he had been working with: 'Milltown boys don't grass' remains a golden rule. He had said this expressly to the judge: "where I'm from, you never tell people's names". He said he had never seen such a glare on a magistrate's face since his teenage days in the 'electric blue' court standing before the stipendiary magistrate (see *Five Years*, pp.59–61).

Danny emphasised that he was not 'proud' of his way of earning a living:

> I've kept going for the kids. When Cathy [eldest daughter] was 16, I was going to stop. Then Ophelia came along, and I was stopping when she was 16, to see her through her childhood. Now Alfie's here. When he's 16, I'll stop. That'll be the end of it. But then probably someone else will come along, so I'll have to keep going[54]!

---

54 Shortly after I completed an almost final draft of this manuscript (in August 2020) I called Danny to wish him a happy 61st birthday. He told me he now had a new market – face masks. He'd already 'delivered' two orders and had another order for 100: "I sell them for £1.50 and you can buy them for £3.00 from the shop; that's not bad, is it? A bit like Robin Hood, somebody's got to do it to help people out when they've got to wear them". The money he had made had already paid for his car insurance, so he could drive Alfie around legally.

That was always expressly the main concern of the Boys – their children, initially, and later, their grandchildren. They themselves did not lead lavish lifestyles. However, their children did, at least in the sense that they 'wanted' for very little; almost every wish was granted and, as I wrote in *The Milltown Boys Revisited* (p.211), they also equipped their kids with the 'gadgetry of competence', the resources and technology that would, somehow, make them clever! Alfie, Danny's five-year-old grandson, has his own bedroom in their house and stays there most weeks: "he's got everything, a real boy's room", said Danny. The rewards of offending are almost exclusively splashed on him. This is the rub. In classic criminological parlance (see Sykes and Matza 1957), the Boys invariably invoked 'techniques of neutralisation' and 'vocabularies of motive'. They blended versions of an appeal to higher loyalties and a denial of victims. Everything they did, they said, was for the family and the kids. The drug dealers said they abhorred heroin and crack cocaine; they just dealt in 'weed' (and in fact, often, also 'speed'). The shoplifters said that they stole from well-known high street chains: if Philip Green (the 'king of the high street') could afford *two* super-yachts, he must have ripped off his workers, so why shouldn't they have a very small slice of that cake? They had a point. Certainly, the income they generated was generously distributed to their children (and latterly their grandchildren) who, as many of the Boys put it, never "wanted for nothing". They were acutely aware of the poverty in which they themselves had grown up, walking around with the holes in their shoes stuffed with a rolled-up newspaper, wearing 'hand-me-downs' from older siblings and so forth, until they had first got odd jobs in Milltown and later, or in parallel, started stealing. That brought some possibility of living 'on a par' with other kids (see Danny's *Rec-Boy* song, above). Their children clearly did not want for anything. I often witnessed the Boys handing out money on request; Christmas and birthday presents were showered on the kids, and now the grandkids. The scale of expenditure on 'the family' was often quite staggering, but lifestyles were otherwise quite modest. I suppose it would have been unwise for many of the Boys to be too ostentatious in their consumption, given that they often appeared to have rather limited visible means of support.

And yet, when they could, taking a leaf out of the gangsters in the films, they liked to 'flash the cash', pulling out a wadge of £20 notes [not £50 notes – that invited too many questions and that denomination of note was often either refused or checked]. Ted, who had moved away from Milltown before he was 20, had established himself on an equally tough estate elsewhere. After Gary had phoned Ted during the Covid-19 crisis, Gary called me to say that it had been good to talk to his 'old mate': "he sounded pretty good about the cancer and up there, How, he's really king of the pile". Gary recounted a mutual acquaintance who had reported the respect with which Ted was held on the estate. I asked Gary whether it really was respect, or rather fear:

> Oh, a bit of that as well, yeah, I know there's that side of him. He can probably still look after himself. I took on a lad from that place, and he'd had a pasting

from Ted over some drugs thing; when he found out I knew Ted, he told me that he thought he was a complete cunt.

Ted would not have appreciated the comment. He liked to think of himself as 'the nicest drug-dealer you would ever want to meet' (see *The Milltown Boys Revisited*, p.51) – and his dealing tended to be very relaxed and amiable (people just dropped by, left the money on the top of a chest of drawers in the living room and took a bag of weed from a drawer; typically Ted greeted them with 'hello, love' or 'all right, mate', though he often didn't even turn around, certainly not when I was there – but he was definitely not like that to those who got in his way or cramped his style. With them, there was a ruthless response; it took a survival of the fittest approach, in that environment, to remain king of the pile.

Mark had been a prolific offender in his youth, though his mother once famously suggested to me that "he would not be in so much trouble if the police did not keep on arresting him"! In his adult life, he has largely avoided contact with the law, particularly since he became a postman (17 years ago). His wife, Veronica, however, committed long-term benefit fraud and when she was convicted she narrowly escaped going to prison.

BENEFITS CHEAT WHO 'NEEDED HELP TO GET OUT OF A CHAIR' CLAIMED £35K WHILE WORKING AS A BARTENDER AND CLEANER

[edited for confidentiality]

A benefits cheat who said she needed help getting out of a chair claimed more than £35,000 in disability benefits at the same time as she was working as a cleaner and bartender.

Cardiff Crown Court heard Veronica _____, 52, received Employment and Support Allowance after stating she needed help to get out of a chair due to severe arthritis.

In her police interview the defendant told officers she did not think she needed to declare the work as it was "only a couple of hours".

The court heard she made the fraudulent claims between 2007 and 2016.

Prosecutors said the claim was legitimate when she first applied for disability benefits in 2003 as she was unable to work due to ill health.

_____ signed paperwork saying she would notify the Department for Work and Pensions of any change in her circumstances that may affect her entitlement.

But she failed to declare that she had started working more hours than permitted under the conditions of the benefit.

The court heard she was working as a cleaner and behind the bar at _____ _____ social club.

Her benefit claim stated she had difficulty walking, could not be on her feet for long, and needed help to get out of a chair.

Prosecutors said the total overpayment was £35,645.40, which was paid into her bank account.

When she was interviewed by police the defendant accepted she had failed to declare that she was working several nights a week.

_____ pleaded guilty to three counts of benefit fraud.

Her defence barrister said she still suffers from severe arthritis and added she had no previous convictions.

Judge _____ noted the claim was not fraudulent from the outset.

She added: "This went on for a long time and amounted to over £35,000".

_____ was handed a 26-week jail sentence, suspended for 12 months and ordered to complete 180 hours of unpaid work.

She must repay the money under the Proceeds of Crime Act.

The responses on Facebook to Veronica's offence and conviction were, predictably, varied but perhaps surprising in that they spanned the spectrum of that predictability. On the one side, there was a fusillade of sympathy and support: Veronica was 'hardly a terrorist'; 'cleaners and bartenders don't have offshore accounts'; 'obviously criminal, [but not] a large amount of money in the grand scheme of things with these scumbag corporations not paying their tax'; 'Nothing compared to tax frauds'; 'Sort the massive expenses fraud out from the MPs, sort out the tax evasion … from the Fatcats … Until then stop hounding the little people who rip off a tiny proportion in order to survive'; 'Perhaps stories about unqualified assessors taking away disabled people's benefits would be more beneficial to the public as a whole'; 'Pick on the billionaires who don't pay their taxes before you pick on someone like her'; 'Good luck to her. Get what you can while you can'; 'So many tax avoiders out there, go run a story on them'; '£3.800 per year. That's only £700 more than what tax avoidance costs EVERY tax payer in the country'.

On the other side, there was unconditional condemnation: 'she should have gone to prison'; 'they are just devious people they wouldn't know a days work if it bit them'; '180 hours unpaid work for claiming £35,645, about £200 per hour – people on the minimum wage would have to work over 4700 hours to earn that'; 'If any of you people, who agree with this cheat, or your family were genuinely disabled and were unable to get benefits, you would be up in arms ranting and raving'; 'Other people are struggling … she wasn't, with benefit and job – decusting'; 'Yet another benefit fraudster been caught, should be made to pay it all back and not at a silly amount like £5 a wk'; 'Disgusting I hope they throw the book at her'; 'About time the law clamped down on the bloody scroungers of society'; 'Why is everyone crying foul. She is dishonest and got caught, end of'; 'She should go to jail'; 'Make her pay every last penny back and stop her benefits for good'.

And so it went on, with hordes of people slugging it out on Facebook, using Veronica's case as the punchbag. There was only one lengthy but informed comment amidst the 60 plus posts:

> Amazing how quick papers are to report this sort of rare event yet they do not report of the thousands of disabled people being persecuted – some to the point of suicide – over unfair biased and constant disability assessments, that are undertaken by badly qualified assessors with dubious medical qualifications. These assessments do not even take into account doctors recommendations and the massive majority of claims are denied, only to be overturned on appeal costing the taxpayer more money than is saved. This sort of fraud accounts for less than 0.05 percent of all benefit fraud (which is a lot less than benefits that goes unclaimed every year just by pentioners alone) … But don't let facts get in the way of demonising a whole swath of disabled people… devide and conquer, that's the rule.

I have dwelt on the case at some length simply because it captures so many of the contradictions that inform perspectives in Milltown and which thread through the Boys' attitudes to most aspects of their lives.

The profiling of this case in the local media had caused something of a rift between Mark and Jerry, despite their close lifelong friendship. Jerry wife, Sam, had been quite irate when she learned that Veronica had been milking 'the system' so successfully for so long, when they had battled for an equally long time to get 'the system' to make better provision for their profoundly disabled daughter Rachael and, latterly, to top-up Jerry's occupational pension. Sam had no particular wish to vilify Veronica but she harboured a deep sense of injustice that Veronica had 'got away with it' – in other words, allegedly living the good life and being allowed to continue to do so – while they had struggled on, staying on the right side of the law, yet seemingly 'punished' for doing so. Sam had been made redundant but was not eligible for any benefits because of Jerry's pension. Meanwhile, despite her conviction, Veronica had held on to her job at the local social club.

Jerry was somewhat more 'sympathetic' after an initial attack on 'the system' for its lack of support for people with disabilities:

> She'd had a very nice car through Motorbility, but we'd struggled to get suitable transport to help Rachael. A Ford Fiesta was not big enough for her wheelchair, but a larger adapted vehicle would've set me back around £27,000. We just couldn't afford that. Veronica's fiddle was a year's decent wages for an honest working man. Mind you, the media suggested she'd fiddled that much almost all in one go, when in fact it was over almost ten years. That's not much more than three grand a year, and then I suppose it doesn't seem so bad. Mark said that Veronica genuinely believed that it was OK just to be helping out down the club from time to time, for cash in hand.

Yet again, we find classical 'techniques of neutralisation' kicking into the narratives of the Boys. Veronica's offence was not quite so bad after all, though Jerry knew only too well that she did not just help out 'from time to time'; it was regular work, albeit off the books.

Mark himself talked through the experience:

What it was, right, is that she's full of arthritis and they know this, from all the doctor's reports and everything else. But she was allowed to work 16 hours a week, and then they called her in, 'cos she'd worked over 16 hours. So she admitted that. It was about three or four thousand pounds she owed. And after that she done everything right, everybody told her that. We never, ever had the money. All we ever had was the car, you know, the disability car. She never, ever said she couldn't do things, only on her worst days, that the doctor knew about. And then when she had this interview with an investigator from the social security, she said well if I done wrong by you, then I must have done wrong by the disability, too. So, in that way, Veronica put her foot in it. So then the disability investigated her and she ended up in Crown Court.

Well she shit herself, 'cos they said we owed 35 grand and all that bollocks, and she was crying her eyes out 'cos she thought she was going to prison. So, anyway, as it turned out, she got six months suspended and they put it in the paper, on the front page, that she was a massive benefits cheat. And you know what people are like, when they don't really know the story, you know what I mean, How ... Well, I don't go on Facebook, but if they can't say it to your fucking face, then I don't want to know. She even warned me that there were people up the club pointing the finger, but I said I'm not bothered about that. Like my father used to say 'names won't hurt you, son, don't bother about people calling you names'. Nobody never said anything up the club. Whether they were saying it behind my back, I don't give a shit.

Anyway, you've just got to get on with things. It was wrong, to me, that they put it on the front page of the paper, like she was some big fucking criminal. But there you are, it's done and dusted now.

She was a horrible cow of a judge. We were supposed to be going on holiday the following week, to Tenerife, where we often go. I'd paid for everything. It was the week after her first appearance and her barrister mentioned this because he wanted her next appearance to be after we come back. 'Going on holiday?', she said, 'what on earth would the public think of that?', and she stopped us going on holiday. So I'd paid £900.00 for the holiday and I lost that. It was *my* money that paid for that, because what she did was nothing to do with me; it was all on Veronica.

And when she was sentenced, given the six months suspended, my boy [son, Colin] stood up and said 'come on then, mother, let's go to the pub', and this judge heard it and told her to sit down, and the judge said 'go to the pub? What do you mean? This is no laughing matter', and I thought, oh God, she's going to fucking send her down now.

> And after that we were in court again for the Proceeds of Crime things
> they put on us, and I had to find 25-grand in six months, otherwise she'd go
> to prison. So I had to get money on the house. I had a financial adviser and
> they got me the money. That's why my mortgage is so big; it cost me about
> £100 a month extra for the next ten years.
>
> It was a bad time for us, but we got through it. You know what they say,
> today's news is tomorrow's chip paper!

Mark's comments are revealing. He projects a range of characteristics that are typical
of the Boys – the sense of a 'fair cop' (in that, once investigated, they hold their hands
up to their offending), the disdain for those who cannot speak up to your face, and
the sense of injustice when arguably extraneous issues are dragged into the picture and
'unfair' consequences result.

Without any attempt at rationalisation or justification, however, Paul recounted his
criminal history to me, starting with the statement that since I last talked with him,
he had 'only' been to prison twice more, though not for the shoplifting offences for
which he had previously typically been committed to custody. He said that he hoped
he wouldn't end up inside again, because these days he knows nobody there any more:

> I know it's all my own fault, How. I've been to prison 15 times, the first time
> when I was 17. All the way through. Like Danny, he was in and out of prison
> more than any of us. So I've done loads of sentences, not big ones, like years
> and all that, but you're getting older and you're still going back. And then you
> start thinking, well I started thinking a couple of years ago, when I done time
> around twenty years ago, I would have been about 38 and thirty years ago,
> about 28, forty years ago when I first got put inside, I was just 18, ten years
> ago, about 48 … well, you're getting older and none of the Boys you'd expect
> to see would be there. You know, there'd be a lot of us in there before, but now
> it's all the young ones that you don't know. And you think 'what am I doing
> here?'; I'm nearly 50, do you know what I mean? Years ago, you'd always see
> some of the Boys you knew, so many people you'd know, but now, they're
> either gone [dead] or they're not getting into trouble no more, so now I'm
> hoping I've done my last sentence because I don't think I can survive in there
> any more …

This echoed an observation Danny had once made. When you first go to prison, as
a young man, you pride yourself on your toughness, physique and fitness and get
through by ridiculing the 'old lags' who have been in and out all of their lives, never
for a moment believing you may end up like them. It is when you have become
one of them, the subject of ridicule by the young men following in your footsteps,
that you *think* longer about 'doing time' and *work* harder on minimising the chances
of it happening again.

Soon after the collapse of his relationships, Paul had been sent to prison for
12 months, though he served just three months because he was released early on

a tag,[55] for dangerous driving (drink driving), but this conviction was unusual, he said. Normally he had gone to prison for 'instrumental'[56] offences: "all my life, I'd do anything to make money". His most recent time in custody, some ten years ago, had been a 15-month sentence, when he was not permitted early release on a tag, so he served seven and a half months, for growing cannabis in his flat:

> Someone came up with a big idea that I was going to end up a million-aire but it didn't go to plan. I was going to grow ganja, so I used my flat or, really, *they* used my flat to grow it, because I didn't really know how. They didn't force me to do it. To me, it sounded like a good idea. And it was … for about 18 months, before I got caught – they'd grow it and take it away, and they'd throw me a few hundred quid. I was happy with that. Well, I was until I got caught! That was the last time I was inside. I really don't want to go to prison again.

Those of the Boys still embroiled in criminal activity of various kinds (these days, usually either shoplifting or drug dealing) recurrently talk about *hoping* not to end up back in prison, but it is invariably 'hope', and they recognise that imprisonment remains an occupational hazard. As Ted would say, repeating the oft-used cliché, "if you can't do the time, don't do the crime".

Danny, whose custodial history is, as Paul noted, second to none amongst the Boys, though it is many years since he has served time, talked about the banter and repartee that prevails between lifetime offenders and those who work in the criminal justice system, whose lives and careers have evolved in parallel with his own. In court appearances, he has possibly avoided custody on a number of occasions through 'fronting it out': when asked if he has anything to say, he has honed a mixture of impertinence, penitence and helplessness, trying to explain away the offence as a maverick moment based on frustration, anger or sadness (usually connected to some mythical domestic row) while acknowledging his awareness that a custodial sentence may be pending. He 'respects' the fact that the (magistrates') court may be considering a six-month sentence, but then points out how accustomed he has been to serving three months (the tariff) – just 90 days! He gets the message across that he is so used to imprisonment that it hardly constitutes a punishment. On that

55 With some exceptions, convicted prisoners typically serve half of their sentence. Those serving sentences of between three months and four years may be released even earlier on a tag. This is known officially as 'home detention curfew'; the electronic tag attached to the ankle enables location monitoring outside the home and compliance with curfew conditions. Research suggests that electronic monitoring "may help some people to break habits and limit opportunities to commit crime, enhancing opportunities for employment and training, and allowing relationships … to develop" (Ministry of Justice/HM Prison & Probation Service, *Home Detention Curfew (HDC) Policy Framework*, April 2020).

56 The very first article I published sought to distinguish between 'instrumental' and 'expressive' offending by the Boys, and sometimes the cross-over between them (Williamson 1978).

account, despite his record, magistrates have routinely decided *against* a custodial disposition in favour of an alternative.

One prison officer started on the same day as Danny's first day in Detention Centre:

> He started with 'you ever been here before?'. I said 'no'. He said 'well you can start by calling me Sir'. No, Sir, I said. He came over with my clothes and told me to put them on and he said 'it's my first day, too', and told me I'd get used to it, and it'd be easier if I just got my head down and did my time. His name was Mr Winstanley.
>
> And as the years went by, and I was in an out, in and out, and there'd always – well not always, but a lot of the time – be Mr Winstanley there. And he'd say, 'look who's back, the one who said he's never coming back, look who's back'.
>
> Then in one prison I was over the main [wing], fifteen years later, and some screw said 'Governor wants to see you' and I asked what have I done and who is it, and the screw said 'Mr Winstanley, Mick Winstanley'. Oh, is it, I said, and I went to see him. He was Acting Governor and he told me he was off to London and I said something like 'fucking hell, so I'd better say good luck, then', and the screws reprimanded me for my language, 'you can't talk to the Governor like that', but Mr Winstanley said 'oh it's alright, we've grown up together in the prison system, he's all right, I just wanted to have a chat before I move on'!

And, on another occasion:

> My solicitor says to me, 'I've got good news and bad news'. I said, 'give me the bad news'. He said, 'you could easily go down for four months today'. I said, 'what's the good news?' He said, 'well I've seen your record and all the bird [prison time] you've done, you'll piss through it, no problem'!!! I think that's why they don't send me down no more; they know these short sentences just don't bother me. You're talking months – not much. If it happens, it happens, you *have to* take it on the chin. You can't do nothing else.

This, however, is the tough and fatalistic side of Danny's talk. Later in the research interview, he elaborated on his *Rec-Boy* song, when I asked him whether he had regrets about the sheer volume of time he had spent in custody:

> No, I've never thought about it, because that's the way to avoid regrets. You know what I mean, if I think about it, I'll have regrets. It just happened. It's done now. I got through it. Like I've told you before, I hated it, but I couldn't show it on the outside. Inside of me I'd be crying. Outside of me I'd be laughing. I remember when I was first sent down, to DC [Detention Centre].

I was gutted. I was more than gutted. But I done it. Never show pain outside, that's what my father always used to say. Keep it inside, so no-one can see it.

I didn't like one day of it. Especially when you have loved ones on the outside. Like Cathy was born when I was doing time. Before all of that, it was easier. When you didn't have a girlfriend to think about, when I was in borstal and in the early days in prison, I could take it more, but it still hurt. It always hurt.

Danny confessed to being a pathological thief:

I am. I can't help myself. I go out, when I don't have to go out, and I'll get bacon, cheese, sausage, meat, coffee, and just put it in the cupboard. We haven't bought stuff like that for ten years or more.

But this is where I've always been genuine. I wouldn't go in your house and ever take anything, however easy it was. Any of my mates' houses. Even in a stranger's house, if they invited me in. But in shops, or a car with the window open ... well that's fair game. But I won't steal off people I know.

I don't know why. It's just the way it is.

Many of the Boys are now completely detached from offending behaviour or even any contact with it. Kelvin had been "one of the originals" – a reference to the two-week Crown Court trial in which seven of the Boys had been charged with assault, affray and malicious wounding with intent. Spaceman had been injured so badly that he had received the last rites and Jamie had also been hurt. Neither of them was put on trial. Of the others, however, faced with imminent imprisonment if found guilty, this experience had been a significant 'wake-up' call for the likes of Gary and Kelvin. Yet Kelvin still does not see the behaviour that led to the charges (for which they were found not guilty) as "really a criminal act", on the grounds that they rarely went looking for it: "at the time, you went into town with the Boys and got into a fight, it's just something that happened to us". He argued, as I had in my first published article that derived from a conversation with Marty in the 1970s (Williamson 1978), that by their late teens, the Boys had already taken two different paths in their offending behaviour:

Obviously, it was breaking the law, but we didn't really see it like that. It was just something that went on. I mean, there were the other Boys who went robbing and stealing. And stealing, well I wasn't much into that ...

I always look at it this way. You're either a criminal like that, out of necessity; you need to steal to survive, or you do it because you get a kick out of it. And a few of the Boys used to go out stealing even if they didn't need the money, and there's no excuse for that, is there.

It's a path you can either go down or don't go down. I didn't need to. But there's a reason why people go down these paths. Well, the two reasons I've explained.

The only thing that really sickened me was when some of the Boys who were stealing from people, were stealing from people who were worse off than them. I don't think any of it is right, but that's got to be worse.

But if it was a necessity, because you were short of things in life, you should still not be doing it to people who've got less than you.

I think we've got to realise that there's things now that we understand about people that we didn't know then. People's mental health and stuff like that, that we can talk about now but we didn't in them days. A lot of the Boys who did do those criminal acts, like breaking into houses, they had problems at home but it wasn't something you talked about. You didn't come out and tell the Boys that your father had just beaten shit out of you, or that you were starving hungry because there was no food in your house – you know, everything was always hunky dory. So there were issues in those days that nobody knew about.

I don't think the kids today who behave like that have any excuse. They've just got no respect. But in them days, there were probably reasons that we didn't really know about.

Since the Crown Court case involving a number of the Boys when they were in their late teens, Kelvin – who readily admits that he 'shit himself' when he was arrested and put on trial – has had no further brushes with the law.

The last time Tony transgressed the law was apparently inadvertently driving the wrong way down a one-way street, though Spaceman suggested to me (we were in the car with him at the time) that it was a small symbolic act to show that he had not shed his punk rebelliousness completely. Tony's social network is now largely, as he put it, "from the professional classes", who join him for a drink or with whom he goes out for a meal. Tony listed some of his current friends – fund managers, non-executive directors, company directors, entrepreneurs: "Of course, I'm a bastion of the establishment these days, but the others do like to remind me that I grew up on a council estate"!

8

HEALTH

Needless to say, the health of many of the Boys at the age of 60 is not great, though it is perhaps also remarkable that so many have survived that long and that quite a few are actually in reasonably good shape. Over the past 20 years, only one of the Boys featured in *The Milltown Boys Revisited* has died. As we know, Marty passed away in 2014. And as this book was being prepared for publication, in January 2021, Ted, too, passed on. It is important to note, however, that many others close to the Boys' networks (and, indeed, within the Boys' networks, but who were not interviewed in 2000) have also died. Mal's older brother, for example, died unexpectedly of a heart attack. As already noted, I learned in the church at Marty's funeral that Buster had died in 2005; he was 1 of the 12 I had acknowledged in my thesis, though I had not interviewed him in 2000. I have also noted already that seven of the Boys who were on my list in 1999 as possible respondents to be interviewed in 2000 were already dead by then, long before the age of 40.

Mortality and morbidity have therefore been around the Boys for quite a while. More often, it has been long-term decline in health – both physical and mental – deriving from unhealthy lifestyles, particularly alcohol consumption, and traumatic experiences in both adult life and harking back to childhood.[57] Tony suggested that most of his close mates amongst the Boys were still doing pretty well but acknowledged that "of course none of us know what's around the corner". Kelvin felt much the same.

---

57 There has been considerable interest in recent years in ACEs – Adverse Childhood Experiences – and their impact in later life: see Public Health Wales NHS Trust (2015), *Adverse Childhood Experiences and their impact on health-harming behaviours in the Welsh adult population*, Cardiff: Public Health Wales. This particular report looks explicitly at the impact of ACEs on alcohol use, drug use, violence, sexual behaviour, incarceration, smoking and poor diet.

Given the massive health risks taken by the Boys in their younger days – not just the daily routines of poor diet, heavy smoking and excessive alcohol consumption but the regular injuries incurred in both leisure time fighting and workplace accidents – it is, indeed, somewhat surprising that most have lived to 60. As Ted noted, having just been diagnosed with incurable but treatable cancer (his daughter, Hayley, asked me to help them fully understand the lengthy letter he had received from the hospital, confirming the diagnosis and mapping out the prognosis subject to various caveats, particularly to do with diet), he had already lived longer than nearly all of his brothers (eight of them, only one is still alive) and three of his nephews, all of whom had died around, or well before, the age of 40.

These observations are being made at a time when evidence is being made public of striking health inequalities in British society, notably a 20-year difference in healthy life expectancy between the poorest and richest regions of the country (The Health Foundation 2020). As Ted pressed on with chemotherapy and then radiotherapy, and increasingly struggled to digest food, he still insisted that he wanted no pity or sympathy; in July 2020, I called him to see how he was and he invited me over, but only on condition that "I don't want you fucking feeling sorry for me".

Some of the Boys have already succumbed to, or gone through, severe mental health problems. Richard, like his younger brother before him, suffers from schizophrenia (as Marty did), and I was not able to interview him, though when he met Gary in the supermarket during the lockdown in April 2020 he had said that he would like to see me again. Gary told me that Richard, once a 'bull of a man', indeed a committed bodybuilder (as his Facebook profile image illustrates), was now a "shadow of his former self, just going around in his own little world". Eddie is in a similar state. Shaun, too, has had a lifetime of depression, yet successfully achieved a university degree in electrical engineering after his marriage collapsed and it left him "with nothing else to do".[58] Vic, though now recovered, suffered a mental breakdown after the collapse of his long-term relationship with the mother of his three children. Pete has been 'up and down' for well over 20 years, with good days and bad days; most of the time he doesn't even answer the phone – "everything depends on the mood I'm in".

Even Jerry, in many ways the epitome of a steady, dependable working-class 'bloke', looking after his family and drinking in the local club, had a mental breakdown that was so severe he was sectioned under the Mental Health Act 1959. He was in his mid-50s. He had apparently "started talking rubbish" one day, according to his wife Sam, and she was sufficiently concerned to take him to the Accident

58 As a teenager, Shaun had noticed that in the credits to Coronation Street, it always ended with 'Based on an idea by Tony Warren BSc'. Shaun always thought that stood for 'British Steel Corporation'! I had told him it stood for Bachelor of Science. He had even commented, in his teenage years, that "one day, I'm going to get one of those", but early parenthood (he became a father at the age of 19), three more children and a significant mortgage delayed that aspiration and achievement until his 30s. He has never used his degree in his working life (see *The Milltown Boys Revisited*, pp.45–46).

and Emergency Department at the local hospital. They had had to wait 11 hours, during which time Jerry had been 'very loud' and had repeatedly squared up to the security personnel when they had asked him to tone down. Jerry took up the story:

> Yeah, I was off my fucking rocker, so she tells me. I was surrounded by about ten security men and put in an ambulance that took me to another hospital where I was sectioned and put in a secure psychiatric ward. They said that I took all my clothes off and tried to give them away because other people needed them more than I did. They let me go after a week and I came home. I still don't think it was that bad, but Sam has told me she was really scared for me …

Physical disability has afflicted some of the Boys. As already noted, Jerry had to retire as a postman at the age of 52 owing to his decreasing capacity to walk and an unsuccessful operation on his legs (and two diametrically opposed 'work capability assessments' by the same company, one privately for The Royal Mail – confirming the need for early retirement because he was unfit for work, and one as part of a state contract for the social security system – denying entitlement to some top-up benefits on the grounds that he was fit for work!). Jerry was not so concerned about the decision; retirement has enabled him to tick along watching TV from the 'man cave' in his ever-shrinking garden, as various extensions have been added to his four-bedroomed private house in a quiet cul-de-sac, enabling both of his daughters to continue living there (see Chapter 9).

By the time Jerry retired, his close friend Mark had also been a postman for a decade, following half a lifetime working on the railways. He had learned to curtail his heavy drinking and get up early to go to work. Despite a serious illness and the need for a colostomy bag, Mark says that he is probably now fitter than he has ever been! He has quit smoking ("I never thought I'd ever give up smoking") and he does not dare risk drinking too much the night before, because he is driving vans at 5 a.m. He said he is usually in bed by 9 p.m., once Veronica has gone to work (behind the bar in the social club). Mark has not considered retirement. He can't afford it, he said, because he still has the mortgage to pay off. Nevertheless, he had been very ill throughout much of last year (2019), though apparently not so critically ill that his insurance would pay off the mortgage:

> We went to Tenerife in 2018 and I wasn't well. I was off my food and not pee-ing properly. It was like an empty hosepipe! So, when we got home, I went up the doctor's and he said I'd got a bad water infection … Then the following day he called me back. It frightened the life out of me; they looked at my bloods and thought I might have prostate cancer. But then the next time I went up there, they said that the infection I'd got could've distorted my results, so it might not be cancer. Anyway, they sent me for x-rays and this young doctor called this older fellow over and they were both looking at the screen, and it turned out it wasn't cancer, it was some disease, and it was

the worst case they'd ever seen, called diverticulitis. And the young doctor, who was Pakistani, he said 'you will need major plugging' and I said 'look, I'm not a dog'.

Mark outlined in considerable graphic detail the nature of his illness and what had been required to put it right:

Basically, I had the operation and they took my bowel away and I've got a colostomy bag. I had three operations in the end. I caught sepsis twice. I was in intensive care. Even the nurses who were on nights used to say 'we used to go home in the morning and we didn't expect to see you in the night'. It was that bad. Even the doctors say to me now, 'you don't seem to realise how ill you were'. I had bags from every hole! It *was* terrible. I nearly give up. If it wasn't for this one nurse, in fact all of them, I can't thank them enough. And this one nurse, she sat with me for three hours. It was when my body just couldn't take any more pain. And she kept saying don't give up now. Stay strong.

I went down to seven stone. My boy was calling me 'E.T.' You've got to laugh through these things, How. All told, I was off work for nearly a twelve month. I was in hospital, all together, for about 160 days, 'cos the only way they could give me the antibiotics was through a drip. It was unbelievable.

This doctor came around one Saturday morning, and he said 'Mark, the microbiology team are jumping for joy' and I said, 'why's that?' And he said, 'you've caught a superbug'. He said it's resistant to antibiotics. And I said, 'well good for them, but what about me?' Yeah, they put me on these antibiotics that I think would've killed a bleeding elephant.

Yeah, it was a really, really tough time. Veronica was coming in, day and night. She really thought I was going to die. I remember when they were taking me to intensive care, although I was delirious, her crying her eyes out, thinking that was it.

And it's still ongoing, but things are getting better. I still have to have scans but after the next one, I should just be referred to the doctor's for blood tests now and again. I'm a fat bastard now, up to thirteen and a half stone!

But yeah, it was dark times.

Mark's illness had, in his terms, "come out the blue"; otherwise, he has always felt pretty good. He has replaced smoking cigarettes with an electronic 'Puffer', and though he is still tempted to "have a fag" when he sees people smoking 'on the telly', he said confidently that "being round people who smoke doesn't bother me at all". Neither does he drink so much anymore, though he has had occasional "paralytic moments", as he put it, notably after going on a club outing to the Races, when on the last occasion he cracked his head open as he came back into his house and spent the night in hospital. Veronica has not allowed him to go on another club outing since. Having sunk numerous pints every night of the week in the past, Mark now has a few drinks up the club on Sunday lunchtime, where he is joined very occasionally by Jerry, and, on his week off, perhaps on an evening out with Veronica.

Matt also continues to recuperate from a life-saving operation to free up an artery in his neck; this has not always stopped him becoming involved in public confrontations with the police, though he says that some different medication has now really helped to calm him down:

> It was terrible, How, I went to the dentist with this gammy tooth and he said it was a serious abscess and I was rushed straight to hospital. I went into a coma, just blanked out, and they told me after that I'd been a fit away from death. They had to operate on my brain and they told me that I might never walk or talk again. But I did. I had the attitude to do it. It was hard work. But I've fought back. I've always fought back! For three years I was on these tablets that made me a psycho. The neurologist told me it was because they amplified my nature! I'm aggressive when I see injustice. That's why I'm always having a go at the police …

Matt suffers from memory loss but is otherwise once again in pretty good physical shape. He suggested the need to secure more 'balance' in his life, noting the irony in the fact that, in the past, he had rarely bothered to take the tablets prescribed for him, except the ones after the brain operation: "ain't that funny, How, all those illegal drugs I've taken in my life, but I won't take legal ones, 'cos I think pharmaceutical stuff ain't no good for the body"!

Danny's diagnosed arthritis in his back, that makes him eligible (like Mack) for a Personal Independence Payment on top of his disability benefits, does not generally cramp his style, either in earning a living (through shoplifting) or having an active outdoor lifestyle with his grandson, even if he does have occasional bouts of acute pain. There have been short spells during his life when Danny has not pursued his preferred modus operandi – a period many years ago with the British Trust for Conservation Volunteers (which provides him with an alternative identity as a retired tree surgeon), the time when he was on a tag in 2017 (see Chapter 7) and, briefly, during the early days of the Covid-19 lockdown, until he developed new ways of 'working'. Danny noted that at these times he had been much more relaxed, recalling a mantra that he has invoked throughout his life about the risks of criminal lifestyles: 'you never know if you're going to sleep in your own bed tonight'. At the start of lockdown (March/April 2000), he told me:

> I go to sleep knowing there's not going to be a knock on the door in the middle of the night and I spend the day knowing which bed I will be sleeping in that evening. It's only then, when I feel so relaxed, that I realise that I've lived my life living on my nerves. No wonder some of the Boys are wrecks …

The possibility of getting put on disability allowances has significant benefits for those of the Boys who operate on the wrong side of the law, and while their ailments are not mythical, nor are they often as pronounced as they officially claim. On top of his arthritis, Danny is also concerned about increasing forgetfulness and some inability to control his bladder, but it is his back problems that genuinely cause him considerable pain:

> Well I get bad days and I get *bad* days, when I can really feel it. And it's not just my back. It's started to get to my neck as well. The doctor said it'll go around my body. But apart from that, I can still run across the road. But I am on the sick. Mind you, I've really had to fight for it. I take all the evidence from my doctor up there but they still turned me down. That's why I had to appeal. I must admit I put a bit of it on, but I am telling the truth, even if I go in with a stick and get up and down from the chair so they can see I am struggling with my back. And they say 'take your time, be careful' and all of that. They put in the book that I was up and down like a fucking rabbit!
>
> See, I had to go to this tribunal for my appeal and I'd written everything down but they wouldn't let me speak. And I had this furious argument with the clerk but they gave me the points and I won my appeal. Well, they said my appeal was accepted; you've never won nothing – they don't want to admit it like that!

Danny had attended his tribunal hearing with his father. Most of the personnel had assumed it was him, not Danny, whose case was to be heard. They went up to him to apologise that they were running a bit late. Danny had had to interject, "it's not him, it's fucking me … it's my case, not my old man's". After the hearing, as they drove home, Danny said that his father had remarked "you could be an actor, the way you performed in there, that was good". Danny did not in fact care about the extra money (other benefits outweighed the financial benefits) that accrued to him as a result of the tribunal's decision: "I just wanted them off my back chasing me for fucking work".

In contrast, Kelvin had declined the opportunity of being put 'on the sick', despite the legitimacy of his health condition:

> I think I'm in pretty good shape, although I've put on weight during this lockdown. Oh, and I'm on medication for life, for an under-active thyroid. See, I gave up smoking 19 years ago. I'd smoked since I was 11 or 12 and my old man warned me not to give up because it would make me feel worse. And he was right! I got lethargic, I put on weight. So I had a blood test and they put me on this Peroxin. Apparently, there's 1,000 different chemicals in tobacco, and they think one of them was sorting me out, so when I gave up, that was when the problems started.
>
> No, I don't do any exercise, but my work can be quite strenuous. I'm on the go all day. I have been walking the dog during lockdown but it hasn't helped keep my weight down!

The only thing I really had was, well I used to lift a lot of weights when I was younger and I've got two vertebrae worn in my spine. I went to the doctors and had an MRI scan and they wanted to pin my spine. So they were going to put me on invalidity and I said I can't afford to go on that. And being a Milltown boy (!), the doctor said he was really surprised and he said, you know, you're the first person ever to turn that down! Yeah, I was the first one not to take the opportunity to go on the sick!

But they did say I wouldn't be able to carry on doing my job, tiling, but as it's turned out, I'm still doing it. So it can't be as bad as they thought. Having said that, I do have problems with my back, now and again, but touch wood, it hasn't been too bad for a few years.

No, I've got nothing to complain about. I think I'm doing pretty well.

Vic, too, doesn't complain and rather revels in posting images of himself on Facebook – sometimes still shots with his grandchildren, but just as often video clips in a Bob Marley T-shirt, smoking a spliff, with reggae pounding in the background. When talking about his emphysema, now medically diagnosed so that now he is officially 'on the sick', Vic said that he uses a pump to help him breathe but he walks everywhere and reckons that, by doing that, he gets in a fair amount of the exercise he should be doing. He does not think he is in too bad a physical condition for someone of his age:

> See, when I was working in the chemical plant, I started getting ill and losing weight, so I went to the doctor's and they said, 'oh you've just got a bad cough'. That's what they'd always told me over the years. So I went back to work, but I was really struggling to breathe, so I went back to the doctor's and they sent me for tests, and I was back and forth to the hospital and they told me then that I'd got emphysema ... I struggle walking and I get out of breath quick but other than that I think I'm still pretty fit and healthy for my age. I look at some guys and I think fucking hell I'm in better shape than them. And I'm still abusing myself, with the fags and the weed ...!

Drug use has, however, generally diminished and the cocaine users in the 1990s are generally no longer snorting a line or smoking crack. Some of the Boys are, however, exceptions to that rule. Nathan, for example, continues to use heroin and is routinely referred to by the other Boys as a smackhead. Matt is not a user any more, but – as reported in Chapter 7 – he did try to make money from the drugs trade, with tragic effects for others and very little success for himself. One or two of the others are also still regular users of speed and cocaine.

Some of the Boys continue to smoke the occasional, or more regular spliff, but substance misuse of most kinds has fallen away. Pete said he never managed to kick the habit and still smokes both cigarettes and weed, "and now I'm diagnosed with COPD because of my bloody smoking, and I still haven't quit smoking, so it's degenerating". Mack had been a habitual user of amphetamines, which had for a time threatened to end his marriage (but he desisted, and he and Andrea are still together); now he liked to "just have a spliff with a couple of pints". And whereas only Jerry, of all the Boys who had formerly smoked cigarettes, had ceased smoking cigarettes at the age of 40, now many of the Boys have done so. Even alcohol consumption has declined, largely because there is less collective boozing on a regular basis. When the Boys meet up 'socially', however, for birthdays, weddings and funerals, their drinking remains quite staggering. I am usually driving, so I'm under no pressure to join in (not that I could ever keep up with them). Those who are not driving sink pints as if there is no tomorrow. There are, of course, exceptions. Spaceman, who joined Alcoholics Anonymous in the late 1990s, remains dry and he proclaims with considerable pride that he has not touched a drop for 23 years. Others have moved from beer to wine or spirits, but most continue to consume quantities of alcohol quite similar to those when they were young, albeit on a less regular or routine basis.

Some of the Boys still have their moments! Jerry, on his 57th birthday, went on a pensioner's outing to a seaside resort, with his profoundly disabled daughter Rachael, organised by the social club. He had started drinking before they left Milltown and carried on drinking all day. When it was time to board the coach for the return trip, the driver would not let them on (not least because Jerry was insisting on bringing even more booze on board); the coach left without them. Jerry settled down to carry on drinking, with some street drinkers nearby. Eventually, he pondered on how to catch a train or bus home but given Rachael's limited mobility, he settled for a taxi. It cost £130.00! Sam was less concerned about the drinking and more about that cost. Jerry refused to appear before the club committee to account for his behaviour and was, as a result, banned indefinitely. Though the ban was later lifted, Jerry's attendance at the club is sporadic; today, he prefers to drink at home.

Spaceman suffers significantly with a range of ailments, from COPD to considerable, though erratic, deafness. He had anticipated his declining health long ago when he used the modest inheritance on the death of his mother to invest in an orthopaedic bed and chair, as well as putting some money aside for a stairlift, when the time comes. He joked that he no longer uses four-letter words, like 'jobs' or 'work', even though he had once made some effort to gain some legitimate employment, but his health problems, amongst other things, always got in the way:

> After art college, I did have a lot of pain. I was suffering from arthritis. But nothing worked, no fucking pills worked. I tried to get a job, but there was the problem of my criminal record. H, I've been out of trouble for 24 years now, but even then, it still held me back. I tried for anything. Jamie said to try his place and I wrote a letter and sent my CV, and *they* told me I was too qualified because of my fucking degree! I was in no man's land. So eventually I just decided to stay as the starving wolf.

And I always had health problems. Going back to my head injuries when I had the last rites. The neurologist says there's little they can do, even though I take a bucket load of pills. I've got epilepsy. Sometimes I still don't know what I'm doing. Some days I'm just on auto-pilot. I've been known to walk out into traffic. It's a wonder I haven't got myself killed.

Amongst Spaceman's core crowd of mates amongst the Boys, however – those I usually depict as the 'catholic' Boys, though not all were Catholics: Tony, Gary, Jamie, Kelvin, Gordon and their wider circle of friends – health has not, so far, been a particular challenge. They all still drink too much, but most have now given up smoking and few take illegal drugs. They themselves express surprise that they continue to remain in good shape, despite the ravages of the past and their continuing self-indulgence in the present.

Jamie conceded that drinking and gambling remain his vices. At 50, he'd had his first "NHS MOT" and was convinced it would reveal something wrong with him. But, to his astonishment, "I'd got away with it". He'd had knee and elbow operations from football injuries, but takes more care of himself these days:

> I drink green tea every morning and have to be a bit careful with my blood pressure, which can be on the high side. I do drink a lot on a Saturday, when I still go out with some of the Boys. We still think nothing of ten pints, when it used to be 13-14-15 a night. But we're not as bad as it was then – (laughs) then we'd have eight pints a night during the week and then a bellyful on weekends! Yeah, a bit too much booze. But otherwise I'm good.

Tony, too, said that he liked a drink (these days, it is a good red wine), and, although he doesn't do any active exercise, except walking, he proclaimed he was OK: "I'm not fit, but I'm not ill. I don't go running or go to the gym, but I do go walking. I'm a fat twat, but there you are". Gary also confirmed that, like most of the other Boys in his immediate circle, he was still in pretty good shape, though he admitted to having sunk very low after the death of his son. It took him about a year to come to terms with what had happened, but now "I'm back to work, hard work, and physically feeling great". He contrasted that with some of the Boys who had spent most of their lives ducking and diving on the dole:

> They're falling apart. I'm often giving them money. I can't turn them down because they're my old, old friends. But they see me around and they beg, they beg me to buy them a couple of cans. I can't refuse, but they're pissed or stoned all the time and some are in a terrible state. Amputations, on sticks. Some are OK, but a lot of those boys … they're old men, How, they're old men …

Mack, as noted above, has had a colostomy bag for 14 years. He described it, surprisingly perhaps, as "the best thing that happened to me", a comment that clearly demands to be put in context:

I thought I had bowel cancer but I kept avoiding going to the GP. The pain was getting worse and worse. Then one day I was rushed into hospital and instead they found a hole in my intestine. That was such a relief … I've been fine ever since …

Indeed, Mack said that, apart from that, he really was fine. A few pints, fewer than ten cigarettes a day, the occasional spliff and no exercise – yet he felt in good shape and looked it, too.

I had not talked to Paul since I interviewed him 20 years ago. Even then, he had a serious drink problem. Having got his mobile phone number from one of the other Boys, I called him to explain that I was thinking about writing another book and wondered if he would be willing to talk to me. At first, he couldn't quite work out who I was:

Sorry, How, I only know one 'Howard', and also the way you talk, but I didn't realise at first it was you. I should have known. Howard, from up the Rec. I'm a bit out of it, you see. I'm not down *The Fountain* anymore, by the way, so I don't see so many of the Boys. I'm living by *The Highbury*. I'm usually in the pub. Not at the moment, of course, 'cos of this lockdown. It's best to call me in the middle of the day, just before I start drinking, even if I might've already had one or two. Not in the morning, 'cos I'm not in the mood for talking then. Just call me about 1pm. If my head's already fucked, I'll tell you. Sometimes I don't know one day from the next one. One day I'm up, the next day I'm down.

Yeah, sorry How … Of course, I'll talk to you. You've always been brilliant with us. I'm just amazed you're still thinking about us, after all this time …[59]

Living on his own, as he does these days, Paul drinks excessively, and continues to consume significant quantities of illegal drugs (mainly cocaine, at £40 a gram), though he rejects the label of 'pisshead', even though he is well aware that others see him in that way. Simultaneously, he claimed that "I know when I've had enough" and "my problem is that I've got no-one to calm me down". Paul conceded that he had been using and abusing various substances all his life:

---

59 Within two hours, Paul had called me back and left a message on my answerphone:

How, sorry to bother you, but I've just been telling these two nice girls about you. One's a psychologist – that's somebody who deal with your head – and she wanted to know more. And then I realised I don't know what your name is. I just know you as Howard from up the Rec. I said you were a Professor, that's right, isn't it, and they didn't believe I could know a professor, so can you tell me what your name is, please …

I sent him a photo of the cover of *The Milltown Boys Revisited*.

I mean, I was on the glue longer than nearly everyone, me and Jerry. I was still sniffing glue when I was 25. It took the shit out of my head. I didn't know I had shit in my head but now, looking back, I think I must have had shit in my head and that was my way of dealing with it. Now I'm just drinking every day. You know when people say 'oh, I don't feel like a drink today'. I *never* feel like that. I have a drink for everything. If I'm feeling good, I have a drink. If I'm not feeling very well, then I have a drink, to make things better. I've got to have a drink before I do anything. I've been doing that for years. When I was working, I'd have eight cans after work and then maybe five pints in the pub, and, oh yeah, whisky chasers with all of that.

With this lockdown, I thought I might control it but I think I've got worse. I stocked up a couple of weeks ago with three bottles of Jack Daniels, a crate of Magners, a crate of Stella. You know, I've been panic buying booze. Booze was my toilet roll! And I drank all of that in a week, so I had to get some more.

So I'm not better, but I can't afford it now, because I'm down to my pennies now, whereas before I had money in the bank. I didn't think about money. It was, just carry on drinking. Now I've just spent my last £15 on a half-bottle of whisky and another four cans. Before that, today, I've had six cans, a quarter bottle of whisky. I started drinking at 10 o'clock and didn't have nothing else. And then I panicked, what if I need a drink later? So I've just been out and spent my last £15.00.

Surprisingly, perhaps, Paul has otherwise had few physical health problems, beyond some benign tumours he had removed a few years ago, and treatment for injuries incurred when he walked out into the road in front of a car. Incredibly, although there was a lot of blood ("because I smacked my face into the windscreen, so most of it was from my nose"), he incurred no broken bones. He does, however, continue to have flashbacks about the accident, though he says he can't really remember what actually happened. This is consistent with a range of other mental health problems Paul has faced throughout his life. He talked about his paranoia that "explodes when I go to the shops", his profound lack of confidence and self-worth, and the confirmed anxiety and depression that enables him to remain 'on the sick', though he admitted that "I do play it up a bit, of course … like every-body does". Once again, he returned to his drinking, saying that it bolstered his confidence and gave him the courage to talk to people, even to me! Without a drink, he said, he would never have sent me a text to say that he was ready for the research interview: "I've had a drink but I'm not hanging; I just didn't want to let you down".

The health of the Boys is evidently not likely to get any better. As I was con-cluding the manuscript for this book, in early September 2020, I received three messages on the same day. Ted wanted to let me know that, in the coming week, he would be having radiotherapy for his cancer, but that he still wanted to talk to me about his funeral. Jamie, who had suggested earlier in the year that he was in rude health, said that he was going into hospital to have some gallstones removed: 'must get rid of nasty Galway stones' he messaged, with characteristic Irish humour. And Spacemen left a voicemail, saying that there was not much point, right now, calling him about the cover design and possible cartoons for the book, because his hearing had 'gone again'.

9

HOUSING

Many of the Boys were still living in the same places they had been 20 years ago. Those 'places' are, of course, very different forms of accommodation, ranging from privately rented rooms and rented council houses in Milltown, through various levels of owner occupation both within and beyond Milltown, right up to Tony's detached residence in a picturesque village on the England-Wales border ("though it's changed a lot since you last saw it; we've done a lot of work on it – extensions, kitchens, bathrooms, garden, garage – but same place, yeah"). Nevertheless, Ted, Danny, Richard, Denny, Ryan, Tony, Alex, Mack, Mark, Jerry, Shaun, Derek, Colin, Jamie, Eddie, Nick, Tommy and Mal have not moved house since I interviewed them in 2000. This is almost two-thirds of the Boys I interviewed for *The Milltown Boys Revisited* and the vast majority of them are still in the same domestic situation, either living alone (Richard, Colin and Eddie) or with the same partners as before. Only Ted is not. He has not moved from his council house under an hour's drive from Milltown, but he is not with the same partner; his current partner lives just around the corner from him in her own house and they move between the two. Of those 18 individuals still living in the same place as they were 20 years ago, 11 are in Milltown (and Marty was, too, before he died), four do not live very far away, two live beyond the city but within an hour's drive, and only one lives a considerable distance away (see below).

Of the others, six have moved within Milltown, one has returned to the estate, and four have moved from one location beyond Milltown to another. But within those relocations, some very different stories can be told.

Kelvin has moved once and, at the time of the research interview, was on the point of moving again – just 600 yards down the road, downsizing from a four-bedroomed to a three-bedroomed house. Technically, he still lives in Milltown, but no longer in the heart of the council estate or in the house he bought through right-to-buy. A new-build estate has been built on neighbouring fields and woodland and

Kelvin moved there in 2002. The house he is about to move to is of the same vintage, less than 20 years old.

Gary now lives on his own in a one-bedroomed apartment in Milltown, though on the other, 'quieter', side of the estate. He bought the flat a few years ago for £80,000. It is a short walk from his former four-bedroomed family home which, like Kelvin's, is also a relatively new-build, on the site of what was once a hospital. The house is still occupied by his ex-wife.

Matt and Spaceman also live in one-bedroomed apartments, though just a short bus ride away from Milltown – Matt in a sheltered housing complex, Spaceman in a strategically acquired flat with roof space to accommodate his paintings and stairs wide enough to take a chair lift which, in time, he anticipates he may well need, given his multiple, worsening health problems.[60]

At Marty's funeral (in 2014), Nathan told me that he had a flat above a row of shops in Milltown, where he had in fact been in 2000, but by 2020 he was precariously housed – "wherever I lay my hat" (which was his response to my question when we bumped into each other in the city centre as he was on his way to the probation office – "where else do you think I'm going, How? Same place as always"). The same was also true of Vic and Nutter in 2020, but Paul, who had been living in the YMCA ten years ago, now had stable accommodation, although he had inadvertently put that at risk not so long ago.

On his release from prison in 2002, Paul had been allocated a council flat on an estate not so far from Milltown, where he had lived for seven or eight years and where he had been persuaded to grow considerable quantities of cannabis, for which he received a 15-month prison sentence:

> So I lost my flat. And I lost all my furniture in it, because I didn't have nowhere to put it. I come out of prison – 15 months, so I done half of that because I didn't have no tag or nothing – so when I come out of prison, I went to the YMCA. I've got family and all that, but somebody told me you'll get a place quicker if you go to the YMCA. So I went there for five months, but five months down the line the council told me I was excluded – is that the word? – because of the drugs thing, which meant I couldn't go on the council list for two years. And I thought I can't stay in the YMCA any longer; it was harder than being in prison, to me. I couldn't stay there for another two years, before I could go on the council list. And then somebody told me about this. I needed 1200 quid, for the place I am now, because it's private, so I had to raise the money. And people lent me money. I got it through an agency, so I don't even know who the landlord is. But I can't go nowhere else now, because I've got a roof over my head. At the end of the day, although I put my name down with the council, I'm not moving. I could

---

60 As noted in Chapter 8, Spaceman had a very small inheritance when his mother died not long after he graduated in 2002; with it he bought an orthopaedic bed and orthopaedic chair, which was also part of that planning for the future.

do, because it'd be cheaper. My rent here is £475 [a month] but I'm on the dole, so the social pays it. Well, they pay £455. It's a two-bedroomed flat, but I'm just a single guy, so every fortnight they take £10 out of my dole to give to the landlord.

Gordon and Miranda have moved from a large terrace Victorian house fairly close to Milltown to a large, more modern, detached house a bit further away on the other side of Milltown, though still less than a 20-minute drive away. Trevor has sold his ex-council house and moved to another house in a private development ('not even ex-council', as the Boys depict such properties) on the edge of the estate. And Pete and Barry, having moved to a villa in Tenerife but bought a small flat in the UK, said they had started to "feel like vagrants" journeying between the two – "three months here and two weeks there, and I've never been a great fan of flying". As a result, they have moved permanently back to the UK. But though they live in a modest apartment not much over an hour's drive from Milltown, they do not go back there, nor does anyone know where they live. On the phone, Pete repeated the point he had made to me in the past, that he had "become very reclusive and I don't have much to do with anyone anymore".

In 2000, a third of the Boys were owner-occupiers, many through the 'right-to-buy' scheme promoted in the 1980s by Margaret Thatcher's desire to establish a 'property-owning democracy'. When the maximum discount was applied, this offered a substantial percentage reduction in the market value. It had enabled at least some of the Boys to get their foot on the private housing ladder with mortgages of £10–20,000 for houses that today are valued at well over £100,000. By 2000, four of the Boys had already abandoned owner-occupation, two through selling up (Derek and Eddie) and two as a result of re-possession (Nutter and Vic). All had been unable or unwilling to pay the mortgage. None has revisited owner-occupation again. Three more of the Boys (Ryan, Danny and Ted) had told me, 20 years ago, that they were contemplating buying their houses but, in the event, none of them did. Living as they do in the heart of the area from which the Boys came (the most notorious part of Milltown), Ryan and Laura have no desire to move but continue to recognise the likely difficulties of selling a house there, should they wish to do so (see *The Milltown Boys Revisited*, p.117). Danny and Ted, for a combination of other reasons, have not taken the opportunity to buy their houses. Only one of the Boys (Mark) has ventured into owner-occupation since 2000.

Just as Eddie, Derek and Vic had done during the 1980s and 1990s, a few of the other Boys struggled at times with mortgage repayments, especially during the recession around 2008 (and, in Mark's case, on account of Veronica's court case and huge fine, as a result of which he had to re-mortgage his house) but, by 2020, most of the Boys in owner-occupied accommodation had now paid off their mortgages. Their mortgages were usually never huge in the first place; it was more a question of whether their employment and income were regular enough to meet the payments required. But nobody emulated Nutter who, in the 1990s, just stopped paying after just one instalment and then lived there for 'free' for three years before the legal procedures were concluded and he was evicted. He has lived precariously ever since.

In contrast, Gordon has a property portfolio accruing from his diverse entrepreneurial activities, while both Gary and Jamie have 'second homes' – the former council houses their parents had lived in and in which they had grown up. Gary inherited his from his parents (who themselves had exercised their right-to-buy), buying out his siblings. Gary's daughter, Simone, lives there with her husband and three children.

Jamie's acquisition of his parents' house was a rather more convoluted process. The house had cost just £13,000 ("it was an absolute bargain 'cos we got maximum discount through the right-to-buy"). The original intention had been for his parents to live there for free for as long as they wished. Jamie had agreed to buy it with his brother – £6,000 each, with the remaining £1,000 from his parents, but for various reasons this arrangement took far longer than anticipated. During the unforeseen delay, his father died and the house was finally purchased just six days before Jamie's mother also passed away. Jamie later bought his brother's share – for £50,000. An agency looks after the house – "it's semi-detached with a long garden" – and the current tenants are through a social housing charity ("so I'm doing a bit of good"). On the Purple Bricks website, just a week before I interviewed Jamie, the value of the house was estimated at £151,000. No wonder it is Jamie's 'safety-net for the future'.

The late-comer to owner-occupation is Mark. He still lives in the same house that he and Veronica rented from the council for many years[61] but, having become a postman 17 years ago, he took out a 25-year mortgage and exercised his right-to-buy:

> The reason I can't really think about retiring is that I've still got seven or eight years to go on the mortgage. Yeah, it was a council house and we had it for … well it was valued at thirty-six and a half [£36,500] and we had it for twenty [£20,000], but obviously I've taken other loans out against it to do it up, and then there was the money we needed for Veronica's court case [see above]. And I just bought her a new kitchen yesterday.

Mark's housing costs, relative to income, are by far the greatest amongst the Boys: currently, he is still paying £800.00 a month.

Jerry and Sam had bought a four-bedroomed house on the other side of the estate long ago, both to make provision and have collateral for their daughter Rachael, who has multiple disabilities. When I visited fairly recently, the house now had a number of extra rooms. It is, effectively, a six-bedroomed house, plus a 'man cave' in the garden. Two extra rooms have been built on the back. This is Jerry and Sam's living quarters (a living room and a bedroom). Rachael, who is now 37, has a

---

61 For almost ten years, however, Mark was technically *not* living there in order to maximise Veronica's benefit entitlements. This was one of the ploys used by some of the Boys, which I wrote about in a section called 'Phantom Separations and Living Apart' (see *The Milltown Boys Revisited*, pp.127–130)

room at the front of the house, adapted for her disabilities, together with a shower room that can be accessed with a wheelchair. Her younger sister Chloe, with her two children (a girl of 15 and a boy of 12), now occupy the rest of the main house. Chloe's boyfriend, Jim, has an apartment nearby. Jerry, who has always engaged in making fascinating calculations when it comes to money, explained:

> Chloe had a house in Milltown. She was paying £600 a month rent. She's got a good job (she's a PA for a health and safety project at the hospital), but it was still a lot, after she split up with the kids' father and had to pay it on her own. So we talked about it and she borrowed £25,000 (against the value of our house) to have the extension built here, for us. And then she moved into the main house. She pays back the loan; it's a lot less than £600 a month! She's basically got the house here – three bedrooms and the living room. We all share the kitchen. Rachael's got her own bathroom. Chloe's got one upstairs. And we've got *en suite* through there [pointing to their bedroom]. And I've got my cave in the garden, with a telly, stove and bar. We just watch the TV in here, I walk the dogs and drink a few beers out there [in the 'man cave'].

Given all Trevor's skilful tactics in negotiating an exchange to a council house with a substantial garden, then immediately exercising the right-to-buy and building a huge garage as a games room for himself and his children (see *The Milltown Boys Revisited*, p.112), it was initially depressing to hear that he had split up with his wife and left. That house had been on the edge of the tough side of the estate. Now re-married, however, he lives in a more desirable area, though still within the boundaries of Milltown, in an owner-occupied new-build house, quite close to Jerry.

For those not living in either owner-occupied houses or privately-rented accommodation, their housing costs are often staggeringly low. Both Ted and Danny pay less than £100 a month for their three-bedroomed municipal properties. That rent has been largely unchanged for years. When Ted tried a 'proper job' for a short time a few years ago, his major complaint was that he'd lost his housing benefit, though his rent was only £94.00 a month. He said he was lucky; many people were now having to rent identical former council houses that had originally been bought up by tenants through 'right-to-buy' but then had been bought out by landlords anticipating profits through 'buy-to-let', who were renting them out for around £500 a month. No wonder people had to rely on housing benefit to live there, Ted suggested.

Danny's modest municipal house, at the end of a cul-de-sac in Milltown, costs £17.00 a week to rent. The décor is immaculate. Everything is colour-matched – carpets, cupboards, wall units, tables and chairs, three-piece suite and walls – to the point where it almost feels like a showroom. You just *have to* take off your shoes when you walk in the front door, for fear of marking the white shag carpet that you can see through the glass partition door to the living room, even when he or Nathalie tell you not to bother. It is pristine, though it had not always been like that, when Nathalie had manoeuvred an exchange from the flat they had been living in before:

> Well I had the flat, didn't I, after I split from Maria. And then I met Nathalie and she got pregnant and there wasn't enough room, with one bedroom, for the three of us. And Nathalie said she knew of a three-bedroomed house that we might be able to swap, and that's where we are now.
>
> I said let's go and have a look and we went there and I said fucking no chance. It was a dump, it was a well-used house. And, to cut a long story short, we lived upstairs for nine months while we bashed it through down stairs. I said let's do it in one hit. I had a few quid saved. We had it all ripped out downstairs, new floors, new skirtings, new architrave, even a new toilet. We asked the council and they let us get on with it – 'can we put in a new toilet … Well, if you want to'. We've spent so much money on the house and we like it here. I hope I die here. I want it to be my last place.
>
> I could've had the house for £19,000, it's sad, yeah, because I had £12,000 in cash and if I'd had a way to buy it, I'd probably have bought it, but then the boom come and it was too late. And I didn't want to have a mortgage. Because of what I do, if I got caught and went to prison, well I'd lose it all, wouldn't I?
>
> I could've bought three houses, the money I was getting at that time.
>
> The important thing is that, although Nathalie did all the paperwork, it was me that signed for the house, so it's my house and she can't kick me out. Not that we've ever really had any arguments and if we did, I would go, but she can't make me go, if you know what I mean. That's been a problem for a lot of the Boys.
>
> Where we are, there's a drug dealer just up the road and there's a drug dealer opposite me, but they don't bother me, so I don't bother them. They know I had a name and I know they get warned that I can look after myself, even if now I have to have help with a bit of wood. I keep that by the front door or in the boot of my car, just in case. But that's only if they threaten me, threaten my family.

When she moved back to Milltown, Danny's daughter was allocated a housing association flat that was 'a complete wreck' and he spent a 'few thousand' of his savings helping her to do it up. Once again, seeing that 'the kids are alright' (to lift a title from a song by The Who) is typically paramount in their mind.

As I argued in *The Milltown Boys Revisited* (pp.99–121), however, this snapshot of housing stability and connection to locality conceals as much as it reveals. The Boys have certainly, for the most part, stayed *local*. In 2000, the picture was much the same as above: 19 of the Boys lived in Milltown, eight more lived in the city not far away from Milltown, and only three lived further afield. What is not apparent, however, is mobility within Milltown, mobility between Milltown and other parts of the city, and within the city. Though only Gordon has moved out of the city to

TABLE 9.1 Housing situation since 2000

	Milltown	City	Further afield	
Not moved since 2000	11(1*)	4	3	18
Moved since 2000	7	2	2	11
	18(1*)	6	5	30

Note: *Marty lived in his flat in Milltown until his death in 2014.

a more semi-rural location (which is not actually so far from Milltown), and Pete has moved from England to the Canary Islands and back again, the other nine 'mobile' Boys have also moved in very different ways – at the more secure end of the housing market, Trevor, for example, has moved 'up and across' (to more desirable accommodation on a more desirable part of the estate), while at the least secure end of the housing market, Nathan and Nutter still struggle to establish a base, Paul took some time get his housing association flat, and Vic currently rents a room in a relative's house, in Milltown, though much of his time is spent at Ted's, some distance from the city and the estate, where Vic is hoping soon to be allocated council accommodation. Within the city, Spaceman has acquired a more desirable flat closer to Milltown, while Matt moved from Milltown, via prison, to sheltered accommodation in the city.

10

BELIEFS

All the rules they make – not just the politicians but the judges as well, and the big businessmen – never affects them. That's all I'll say about politics.

(Danny)

Few of the Boys held strong political or religion convictions, though there were some exceptions who certainly had forthright opinions. In their youth, many of the Boys had physically connected with both (extreme) left and right – both the Socialist Workers Party and the National Front – but this was largely for the social events (including physical confrontations) and parties that they offered rather than the beliefs they peddled and promoted.

As they got older, the Boys either shed such beliefs altogether or settled into fairly essentialist positions, peppered with a strong dose of cynicism. Spaceman, who acknowledged that his youthful approach to politics was "casual, naïve and idealistic, you know, everyone should have decent jobs and we should get rid of homelessness – just a dream, really", quoted The Who in response to my question as to whether or not he was still interested in politics: "Meet the new boss ... same as the old boss ... Won't get fooled again". He said that his politics had always been "a bit of a façade":

I've always voted ... always Labour. I say I'm a socialist but then I used to say I was a Maoist ... (laughs) because I liked the uniforms, you know, those tunics with the red stars. I was into the image, not the 5-year plans! Just the image, not the nitty-gritty.

Spaceman suggested that his politics was his sense of fun: "just to wind people up, you know, anti-Thatcher, anti-Boris". He went on, however, in a more serious vein:

I have to admit that I am still in a state of shock that Boris Johnson is the Prime Minister. Since December 13th last year [2019], I've been stunned … that my fellow humans have voted for such a prick. How can people actually believe this shit? It's a form of traumatic stress for me. What, with the Camerons and Osbornes – horrible, thoughtless, heartless, self-serving … Every time I walk past a derelict factory, I think of Thatcher and then I think of this lot … only in it for themselves. We need decency for all of humanity … at the moment, ventilators and hospital beds, not fucking missiles.

Cynicism about 'self-serving' politics ran deep in the veins of the Boys, even if few were as informed or reflective as Spaceman. Danny readily admitted that he knew very little about it and had never voted, but he still had things to say:

Look at the bedroom tax. And I'm not just saying this because they got me for it! But when they had the bedroom tax, this judge said you couldn't put another tax on the council tax. So, what do they do? 7 am on a Sunday morning, they open Parliament just to go in and raise council tax by 20%. And that was the loophole. There's always loopholes.

And the woman who had an oxygen cylinder in her spare bedroom and she still had to pay the bedroom tax, because some judge said she had to, some judge who was born with a fucking silver spoon in his mouth.

They're talking about taking free TV licences away from the over-75s. That broke my old man's heart! But the point is, it won't affect them. They've always got the money to pay.

And this week, some bloke in the civil service,[62] didn't get on with Boris Johnson, so he's had to step down and he's getting a quarter of a million pounds handshake. And he'll walk into another job in no time; he'll be earning 100-grand somewhere else.

Danny readily professed to not understanding Brexit, except insofar as his mother had said Britain had once not been in the 'Common Market' and had been 'OK' then, so probably will be again: "So I wasn't that bothered, really, although now it's like Covid's killed Brexit, 'cos you don't hear much about Brexit any more".

Spaceman warned against talking politics with the Boys. Most were not interested and the rest were either completely with you or completely against you. Ted said he was "staunch Labour", reminding me that he had once been in the Young Socialists and had attended some of their rallies, and said that he still voted "now and again". But he was on the side of Brexit, maintaining an anti-immigration stance and arguing that "only the needy should be let in" because those who were born in the UK were at risk of becoming a minority, and it should be "our country". Jamie was

---

62 This was Sir Mark Sedwill, the Head of the Home Civil Service and national security adviser.

also staunchly Labour, a die-hard 'working man' who had always voted, but who was on the other side of the Brexit divide:

> Labour through and through. What else can I be, How? On Brexit, I voted to stay. We're stronger, better together. That's always got to be the case. The world has gone bonkers, with Farage and Boris. The bus,[63] that poster [Breaking Point][64] – the lies, the scares, the racism. Hard to believe. But in the pub, I avoid the subject.

No wonder. Gary, very close mates with Jamie, had voted *for* Brexit, despite his proclaimed 'love' of all kinds of people and keen interest in current affairs:

> I just love meeting people. Round the world, I just go into bars and have a drink and talk to people. I've met all sorts. It's incredible. I've worked a lot in London. You've got Africans, West Indians, people from everywhere. You know, there was that thing with Stephen Lawrence. Fucking terrible. We're all people together. I'd always read the *Evening Standard*; it's free outside the Tube. I like reading the papers, keeping up with the news …
>
> No, I don't vote. But yes, I'm a solid Brexiteer. You know, they talk about that Windrush generation. Well since then we've been open to every Tom, Dick and Harry – rapists, murderers … We need our borders.
>
> I know they come over to work in bars and they're paid peanuts. It's cheap labour. But they're happy, buying up our houses. They're punching the air, sending money home. Five pound an hour and they're buzzing.
>
> Meanwhile our boys can't get a job. The wages I was once paying them; they were weekend millionaires. They'd get their wages on Friday and they could be on the piss the whole weekend. Builders were catching up with the suits. But with the EU [freedom of movement of labour], wages are dropping like a bomb. Things don't look so good any more for the British working man. That's what we've got to think about. So, I'm happy to give Boris a chance, even though I still won't vote.

---

63 The official Vote Leave campaign used a red bus to promote the message that leaving the EU would leave the UK with £350 million a week to spend on the National Health Service. It was a persuasive but infamous claim, overlooking the rebate that the UK gets back from the EU. Factcheckers suggest that a more reliable contemporaneous figure would have been £234 million pounds a week. Leading Leave campaigner Boris Johnson, later the Prime Minister as the UK exited the EU, was reprimanded by the UK Statistics Authority for the misleading information.

64 During the referendum campaign ahead of the vote on whether or not the UK should leave the EU, in June 2016, the United Kingdom Independence Party (UKIP) launched a poster depicting a column of migrants heading for the UK. It was differentially described as 'controversial' and 'unethical'; the *New Statesman* suggested that UKIP leader Nigel Farage's anti-EU poster depicting migrants resembled Nazi propaganda and described the poster as 'UKIP's lowest point in its campaign for Brexit'.

Kelvin, like Gary, a self-employed and hard-working man, had also voted for the UK to leave the European Union in the Referendum of 2016, despite proclaiming "No, I've never really been a political person":

But I do have an opinion, even if I'd be the first to admit that I don't really understand a lot about it, because I don't go too deeply into thinking about it. But I'll be quite honest with you, I was *against* the EU, I was *for* Brexit. Sorry! There were quite a few reasons put forward that I agreed with. Some of them I've now changed my mind on a little bit, but one of the main reasons was because it wasn't what we originally signed up for. We signed up for the Common Market. And where it had escalated to us being told what to do by another parliament or another government in another country, in Belgium or Brussels, or whatever … well, I just couldn't get my head round it. It wasn't about the Common Market any more, it was about *everything*. It was about a United Europe. That's what I couldn't get my head round. Whereas a common market, where we could trade without restrictions and without red tape, well that made sense to me. But when it came to changing our laws.

And I was bothered about people migrating into Britain in the quantities they did. Not because of any racial issue but down to the fact that … – now don't get me wrong, a lot of the people coming into the country were doing good, for health, the NHS, hospitality sector, hotels, but it also brought a lot of criminals, especially from eastern bloc countries that had joined the EU, and I just thought that was wrong. That we couldn't keep them out. That we couldn't even check on them, on their past. I mean, there was that Lithuanian who killed a girl over here and he'd already done it in his own country and went to prison for it. And they didn't even know! He could walk into this country with his European passport and Britain wouldn't know anything about it.

So, these were the things that I didn't understand and bothered me. I had no qualms with people coming over here picking fruit or working in my industry or in construction, even if I might have moaned a bit about the fact that, yeah, pricing did go down because contractors could get cheaper employment out of those people. But I've never had a go at anyone who was a hard worker. Mind you, I do get annoyed when you hear of those immigrants taking advantage of our social security system, screwing the system, and getting income and housing through us. Yes, I voted for Brexit because I believe we have to govern ourselves and the worst thing is that we still haven't properly left …

I have thought about it more since that vote, because there are things we are going to lose, but I still think we should come out, because we've lost control of our laws and our borders. We should have gone by now. I don't blame Theresa May. I know she was accused of dillying and dallying. But she didn't get shafted by the Europeans. She couldn't get it done because of our own bloody MPs, because they kept hinting that we might still not leave. It was them that knackered us leaving with a good deal. It's been like a game of poker. The Europeans must have been pissing themselves laughing at us, because we showed them our hand. And that gives them the chance to bleed us dry. It shouldn't have been like that. If you have a democratic vote, whether right or wrong, then get on with it. I mean, if we'd voted to stay in, it would've been done and dusted almost immediately, with none of all this faffing about.

Mack, too, was an ardent Brexiteer. He had supported UKIP and voted to leave the EU. He had become more and more angry about "people trying to reverse the decision". He didn't really have any cogent defence of his position or perspective. Mack had voted all his life, for Labour until the 2016 Referendum. In December 2019, he had voted Conservative for the first time, believing that 'Boris' would "stick up for us better than any of the others".

Mark, a 'working man' through and through, had also voted Conservative for the very first time in December 2019. He declared that he really was not very interested in politics, though he had usually voted in national elections (not local ones: "can't be bothered") and, until the last time, always Labour. He had voted Conservative, however, "to get this bleeding Brexit thing done", though his reasoning for leaning that way was somewhat confused and had absolutely *nothing* to do with immigration. He had voted 'Leave' in the Referendum:

> I voted out, I've got to be honest with you. Why should we be sending all those millions abroad when it just seems to get wasted? We've got enough poverty in our own country. You see children starving in Africa. Now don't get me wrong, I feel sorry for children like that. But you've got to stop them breeding, man. Those days have gone. They've got millions of kids and they're always going to be in poverty. We've got to stop chucking money at them. They've got to learn. I mean, *we* were all big families, but nobody can afford to do that anymore. We've got to use our money for us.

I surmise that, in this rather muddled position between the European Union and overseas aid for Africa, Mark was making some implicit reference to the memorable red bus in the Vote Leave campaign: "we send the EU £350 million a week, let's fund our NHS instead", though Mark did not mention the EU in the research interview. Instead, he moved on to make unsolicited comments about the George Floyd street protests and to reveal his rejection of racism (see below), indeed expressing his deep gratitude to the medical and ancillary hospital staff of minority ethnic backgrounds who had cared for him during his serious illness (see Chapter 9), and noting the many cultural backgrounds of those with whom he worked. Immigration was definitely *not* a factor in Mark's decision to vote Leave:

> No, no, Howard, I mean, we've got Polish, Latvians where I work, no, no, that don't bother me. Oh, God bless, Howard, I had Filipinos looking after

me, nurses, and they're the best people ever, you know, without them, where would the health service be? And the bloke who served the food, he was West Indian, and there was another one who did the food, he was Portuguese, and I could always get the food I wanted from them ... Bless them all, without them, where would I be?

Mark had always put his cross against Labour in elections until the 'shambles' of Brexit: "I said to Veronica, I'm going to vote Conservative this time and then I'll never vote again". His view was that all political parties were incompetent but, equally, they were always able, through taxation, to squeeze the 'working man'. And he had always been squeezed by taxation because he had always worked. Whoever was in power found ways of taking money from him "and yet the lazy bleeder next door gets everything". In this way, Mark was echoing Chancellor George Osborne's austerity mantras in the years following 2010 about 'strivers and skivers' and 'workers and shirkers', a rather paradoxical observation given that Mark's wife has been convicted of benefit fraud (see Chapter 8), yet with a strong ring of truth in view of the fact that Mark has worked almost continuously throughout his adult life, unlike many of the Boys around him.

In contrast to Gary, Mack or Mark, Tony was an ardent 'Remainer' and had, for many years, been a committed supporter of the Labour Party, actively campaigning for Tony Blair in 1997 and backing him throughout his tenure as Prime Minister "until things he cocked it up, with the [Iraq] war and God". Now, like Mark, echoing Mark's self-image as a hard-working man, and in tune with Boris Johnson's effective slogan that won him the 2019 General Election, he just wanted to 'get Brexit done'; as a result, Tony, too, had voted Conservative in the election of December 2019 and indeed the time before as well:

> I'm centrist, me. Very much centrist. I hate too left-wing. I hate too right-wing. And that means I can float, then, between different parties. I would *never* have voted for Jeremy Corbyn, never, ever, in my life. Far too left-wing and I think totally out of touch with real working-class people. That's why all those red wall constituencies kicked Labour out. Working-class people are, by and large, patriotic. By and large, they realise you can't have something for nothing. By and large, they don't want to give handouts to people who can't get off their fucking arse themselves. And I don't think Labour really under-stood how deep the Brexit thing was in working-class communities.
>
> I voted to Remain, by the way. But now we're out, we must get out. We need to be nimble now. But I do worry about this government of Boris Johnson's. There's not a single front bench MP in the Tory Party that impresses me, except perhaps this Chancellor, Sunak, but the rest of them are just a bunch of fucking wankers. Labour? In the short time he's been there, I think Starmer is doing a decent job. He's a bit short on personality, a bit bland, but he's doing OK. So far. Bottom line, it's a better-looking Labour Party now.

I was involved locally in getting Blair in. He knew how toxic the Labour Party could be when it got too extreme. I was a big fan of Blair.

I've always voted, and I've moved around. I voted Thatcher all those years ago, because I hated the previous left-wing government, then Blair came along and I connected with him, and then he was gone and replaced by Momentum and Corbyn. So, in the last two General Elections, I've voted Tory. Good luck to Corbyn – get back on the backbenches and have your conversations with Hamas and the IRA. He doesn't really come across as patriotic, does he? Although I do think he is a pacifist. I do think he wants to promote peace.

Many of the Boys didn't vote. Matt said he had *never* voted. Nor had many of the other Boys. Like them, he saw no purpose: "it won't change anything; it won't make any difference".

Paul was a bit of a paradox. My research interview with him took place during the furore over whether or not the Prime Minister's chief adviser Dominic Cummings had broken the lockdown rules and should resign or be sacked. Paul said he had never voted in his life, but volunteered that he 'loved' *Question Time* on television: "it's on at 10:40 on Thursdays on BBC 1; I never miss it", he let me know:

> I like to hear them talk about things, the arguments, the way they always ask questions and challenge what people say. And this Cummings thing … well, it's simple really – you don't need to drive 30 miles to see if your eyes are working or not. That's complete bullshit. *Answer the fucking question.* I never used to like Piers Morgan, but I do now. He puts those fucking lying politicians on the spot. They never answer the questions, do they, they just go round and round the houses.

There are many similarities in relation to the Boys' views on religion. Most of them have steadily 'lost' God over the years; not one has 'found' God. Gary described it firmly as a matter of evolution, introducing his perspectives with "Science every time, H, no religion". He said he had regularly attended Sunday school, like many of the Boys, but this was simply what people *did* in those days, and as soon as he did not have to go, he stopped. His former wife, with whom he remains on very good terms, has always been a believer, but not Gary: "no, H, I was never into God; if it works for others, no problem, but it's not for me".

Jamie had been an altar boy and had rather liked dressing up in smart clothes to go to church. Then, at the age of 13, he decided not to go any more. It had been his choice, he said; and he took an identical stance with his own children. Like Gary's ex-wife, Jamie's wife is still a believer and goes to church every Sunday. They had brought their children up as Catholics but let them have autonomy as to whether to carry on in the faith in their early teens. Neither chose to do so, though his daughter Roisin, who is currently engaged to a "nice lad from the other side of the city", is intending to get married in a Catholic Church. Kelvin, like Jamie, had also been an altar boy, but said he had "no opinions at all" about religion. In recounting how his children, like him, had been educated in catholic schools, he did concede, however, that he had "hypocritically used religion to have a better choice of schools". Kelvin's wife, Julie, is a Protestant, but he still holds on to a modicum of Catholic belief:

> Yes, I believe in God, a bit. I mean, I was brought up that way. And I suppose I'm a bit afraid ... just in case. I know that most of the bad things in this world are caused by religion and so I've never really pushed it. I don't go to church and I've never imposed it on the kids. But for me, well, yes, just in case!

Nine of the Boys in *The Milltown Boys Revisited* had attended the catholic school, five of whom – Spaceman, Tony, Gordon, Jamie and Kelvin – have remained very close friends (the others were Marty, Eddie, Mack and Nutter). Tony made the important distinction between going to a catholic school and being of the Catholic faith. He pointed out that his grandparents ("who were Paddies") were Catholics and he thought his mother was also a believer. He speculated, however, that she had sent him to the catholic school less for its beliefs and more "because it was a better school; if I still lived there, I would've sent my kids to a church school, because they're generally better schools":

> But I'm not religious. In fact, I think I'm a full-blown atheist, if I'm honest with you. Totally. You know, I had a beautiful text the other day, with three pictures: of the Koran, with the words Evidence Mohamed/Allah exists; of the Bible, with the words Evidence Jesus/God exists; and of a Spiderman magazine, with the words Evidence Spiderman exists ... And that's the truth! So, religion, no, if people have got ... and I don't mean stupid, fundamentalist beliefs, but if people like to go to the Mosque, or to Church, or to the Synagogue... I've got no problem with people having faith, but, come on, religion's been responsible for a lot of problems in this world.

Along with others, Matt had long ago abandoned faith, though atypically he had once gone through a period as a 'preacher man', embracing Rastafarianism and walking around Milltown in long robes, with a staff and crowned with dreadlocks.

The non-Catholic boys, like Gary, were almost universally sceptical about religion, turning up, if at all, as Mark put it, "to funerals and weddings, these days in that order". The scepticism of the Boys was captured particularly well by Paul:

> I was brought up a Protestant, but not really seriously. I think you're all entitled to your own religions and I suppose you do have your moments, like when I lost my parents but, at the end of the day, my view is that there's no light at the end of the tunnel. When you're gone, you're gone. Mind you, I'll

say sorry for what I've done, just as my eyes are closing, so if there is a God, I've still got a chance!

Like Kelvin, Paul was also keeping his options open as far as possible, as the Boys always tried to do! Danny was a bit more of a believer than most of his closer associates:

> I believe in God, to a certain extent … if there is a God … Well I've asked Him loads of times, I've looked up and thought of Greg [uncle] and my brother [who died young], and friends … What doubts me, though, is all the wars and famines and volcanos. I know some are man-made, but volcanos aren't, so why would He let things like that happen. And somebody told me something that's always stuck with me: 'if you don't believe, you don't get in when you get there', and that scared me a bit. So at least I can say that I did believe, but what put me off was the earthquakes and volcanos, the bad stuff that happens on the earth.
>
> I know all about the Bible, because you had to do it in all those institutions I was in, well you had to listen …

Many of the catholic Boys were, however, quite fervent in their hostility to faith, though, as we have seen, some have continued to believe, albeit usually at a fairly superficial level. Their antipathy derives from direct or communicated experiences of abuse by catholic priests, not always of the very worst kind (that has attracted significant media coverage in recent years) but sufficient to imbue doubt about the teachings of the Catholic Church. The Boys had been sworn to secrecy, terrorised and intimidated by the very people their parents had told them they had to respect and trust; hypocrisy was the word they typically uttered when talking about this.

Some of the Boys, across denominations, when they had school-age children, had, nevertheless, feigned faith affiliations in order to give their children a better chance of getting into denominational secondary schools that had better reputations. As far as the Boys were concerned, it was just another game to be played in order to secure some advantage in their lives.

Rather more poignantly, almost pathetically, as I talked with him about religion, Spaceman quipped that Marty, through his delusions brought on by schizophrenia, had sometimes thought he *was* God.

11

LEISURE

Danny has only been abroad once, to Spain on a package holiday. He didn't like the smell and found it boring. Jamie has occasionally had a holiday in Greece, including quite recently with his grown-up children, but that's the only time he's ever been abroad. Some of the Boys, in contrast, have travelled quite regularly to many corners of the globe. Jerry has visited some of the wonders of the world. Others head abroad on package holidays. Mark regularly goes to exactly the same spot in Tenerife, together with Tommy and Mal, and Tommy's younger brother, and their wives: "yeah, we all go together, except the year the court stopped us going" (see Chapter 8). Mark and Veronica did take one exotic holiday to the Dominican Republic, to attend his brother's wedding and then to "take a look around". And, although Gary said that he'd "never really been one for holidays", he has seen quite a lot of the world:

> I just love travelling. Travelling for work and travelling for leisure. It's all about the people. The work I do [painting and decorating] has put me in touch with all kinds of people. They know me and I know them. Conversations – that's what life's all about. I've been all over the place. Sao Paolo, Johannesburg, New York. Cities. They're fantastic places. So many different people. I just walk into a bar, and start talking to people. It's incredible. All good stuff, H, all good stuff.

Most of the Boys, however, stay quite local, often spending their leisure time at home. Ted, though he had often been on holiday to Turkey or Thailand in the past, has more recently just sat quietly at home and smoked weed; Vic consumes You Tube videos about black oppression and identity.

Music still figures prominently in their lives, and remains the music of their youth – Bowie, the Electric Light Orchestra, Rod Stewart and Bob Marley. Almost across the board, there is a love of the softer strands of the 'punk rock' music that was the soundtrack of their youth (including early Blondie, such as *Rip Her to Shreds*, and The Police's *Roxanne*), the 'ska' music of The Specials, The Beat and Madness, and the 'mod' sounds of The Jam, although the Boys' musical recollections and current collections are eclectic. They include a strong smattering of soul and Tamla Motown, such as *This Old Heart of Mine* by The Isley Brothers and *What Becomes of the Broken Hearted* by Jimmy Ruffin, through reggae, to some serious rock music, as well as hybrid tunes like *Miss You* by The Rolling Stones. Even older folk and pro-test music, and ballads, were not completely ruled out! Alex now has over 50 Bob Dylan CDs – "nearly the whole collection".[65] Gary recently bought *Jealous Guy* by Roxy Music.

Quite a few of the unemployed, under-employed or deviant Boys had once played quite lot of golf ("it was easy sorting out the drugs on the golf course"), though few did now. Most conducted their leisure time outside of the home in bursts, rather than routinely congregating in the pub (different pubs), as they once did.

It has been many years since Spaceman had a job and, as Jock Young (1971, p.128) noted assertively, "pleasure can only be legitimately purchased by the credit card of work". Young argued that leisure and work are intimately bound together, not watertight compartments, and that, in contemporary societies, individuals were only justified in expressing hedonistic 'subterranean values' (see also Matza 1964) if, *and only if* (my emphasis), they have earned the right to do so by working hard and being productive. Spaceman – an addicted hedonist one way or another throughout his life – would not be so sure, saying that he did not really think about the diffe-rence between 'work' and 'leisure':

> I'm an artist. When I'm awake I'm either thinking about painting, or painting. I sleep and I'm awake. My body clock works best when I get up around 12 and go to bed just after midnight. I just start slowly but by 9 or 10 I'm in full flow, sketching, painting. Of course, I do other things, like go to the football. And I'm always listening to music – 'Should I stay or should I go?' – like The Clash and The Sex Pistols (laughs). Not everything can be found at the end of a paintbrush!

---

65 In June 1978, Bob Dylan was going to be making his first appearances in the UK for 12 years. On the weekend the tickets went on sale, in February, I was scheduled to give a lecture at the Institute of Criminology at the University of Cambridge. I knew the Boys would be in town, so I asked four of them (not Alex) to queue up and buy me four tickets (they were £6.50; I gave them £30.00 – each got a pound for doing me the favour). The Boys hid sleeping bags, a pack of cards and an alarm clock in the park and, after clubbing until about 2 am, they joined the queue, very close to the front. Alex stayed with them. By morning, the queue was three miles long! Alex had never heard of Bob Dylan but thought it might be an idea to buy himself a ticket. He spent the next four months familiarising himself with Dylan's back catalogue and most recent album, *Street Legal*, round at my house, then came with me to London to see Dylan at Earl's Court. Dylan's performances are fickle and unpre-dictable but the Tuesday night was excellent. Alex has been an ardent Dylan fan ever since.

For Spaceman, the punk era remains ascendant, as if it was yesterday, although clearly it is not, as was evident from two photographs he posted quite recently on Instagram. One was from the early 1980s, when Spaceman had been friends with the singer in a moderately successful post-punk band called The Young Marble Giants,[66] who formed in 1978. The picture is of him with Alison, the lead singer, where Spaceman is attired in black leather trousers and he has a full head of short, spiky, black hair. The much later picture of them together was taken in 2017, when they bumped into each other at a gig. She is now a chiropodist; he is attired in flat cap and silk scarf, still with a manifest sense of style. The comment attached to the two photographs is 'Fuck where did it all go to?' The tag to the Instagram post is, interestingly, 'milltownboyz'.

Most of the pubs in Milltown have closed down (Spaceman's 'political' take on this was that it was a middle-class conspiracy to prevent the working-class from organising themselves!). *The Wayfarer* has long been a youth and community project (the irony there is that, when it was pub and came to be frequented by the Boys, the older regulars would complain that it was turning into a 'youth club'). *The Centurion* is now a restaurant. *The Fountain* has been converted into flats, as has another nearby pub. It would now be impossible to substitute the railway stations for Milltown pubs on a home-made Monopoly board; there are no longer even four pubs, when there used to be twice that number, together with a substantial number of social clubs (formerly 'working-men's clubs'). The heavy drinkers in Milltown (like Paul) now crowd into the diminishing number of venues and, almost inevitably, territorial and alcohol-fuelled confrontations ensue. The social clubs that remain and have always been something of an alternative (drinks are considerably cheaper, for a start), but many of the Boys, unlike Mark, don't much care for their regulation and tradition. More and more of the Boys who, in the past, routinely frequented the pubs and/or the social clubs now prefer to stay at home. Trevor certainly does:

> No, I don't go out much – it's too much hassle in pubs these days. Everybody wants to take you on. Too much trouble. And the social clubs are for old men watching the telly and women playing bingo. I might be the same physical age as a lot of them, but I've still got a more youthful mind-set and prefer a drink at home with some home entertainment. It's a lot cheaper as well!

Gary concurred, saying that when he was 'home', he rarely ventured out for a pint in Milltown: "there's too many stupid young fuckers who want to pick on a tall skinny cunt like me". There are anyway, as noted above, not so many pubs to choose from, as Danny observed,

---

66 The Young Marble Giants released two albums: *Colossal Youth* on Rough Trade in 1980, and *Live at the Hurrah* on the Cherry Red label in 1994.

Yeah, for years I was always down *The Fountain* at dinner time, after I'd come back from work. All the Boys were down there. And I'd go down for one or two in the early evening, but I was usually in bed by 9 pm. I have to get up early! But *The Fountain*'s shut and *The Merlin* over the road, so there's not really anywhere to go any more. So, generally, I just stay home, watch quite a lot on the telly and ask Alexa to play some music, unless I'm out with Alfie [grandson], over the woods or down by the river. Otherwise, it's just smoking a bit of draw and watching the telly … I don't see the Boys so much anymore.

Danny admitted he really didn't like venturing out of Milltown, except for 'work'. He does a bit of camping with his grandson, and, as I concluded interviewing him in July 2020, his partner and daughter had just booked a weekend 'glamping', not far away from Milltown. Nathalie and Ophelia also often went for a summer holiday to a caravan on the coast, but Danny doesn't join them: "I don't do caravans".

Others have found alternative drinking venues, both in Milltown and beyond. Denny sometimes goes to *The Vulcan* just beyond Milltown, where Kelvin and Jamie are regulars on a Saturday night. Mack, for example, along with Colin, now frequents Milltown's British Legion club and sometimes goes to *The Highbury*, where he sees some of the other Boys, Paul nearly every time and sometimes Vic, but he is not so keen on going there: the pub is in "enemy territory", in other words on the other side of the main road that cuts the estate in half. Those from the north – the inter-war part of Milltown – have always been hostile to those from the south, which was built in the post-war years and which many of the Boys do not accept counts as Milltown at all!

Paul, however, a former regular in *The Fountain*, has been drinking in *The Highbury* since getting a flat on that side of the estate. In the absence of much contact with the Boys, he met a lesbian couple in the pub and told me that they are now the "life and soul" of his existence. He also made a point of asserting "I don't like calling them lesbians, I call them my lady friends and I love 'em to bits. One's a social worker, like a psychologist, who deals with people in my situation anyway. The other one's got her own cleaning company". Paul sees them quite a lot, not only in the pub. They cook him meals and he said that they seem to enjoy him sharing his stories with them. Occasionally he visits his sister in the Channel Islands but, other than the pub and TV, he doesn't do much, saying that he would like to read books but "my brain won't take me there". In prison, he had absorbed history books – "so long as they had some pictures; you can focus more when you're banged up" – and he watches history programmes on the television.

Jamie, who lives a short way from Milltown, drinks in *The Vulcan*, close to his house. Half a dozen of the Boys "and a few others, a lovely crowd, our age and up to about 73" meet there every Saturday night:

Yeah, we have a few pints in *The Vulcan* and then a few of us – these days, just four or five – go on to town. It used to be about 20: our 'gang', a lot of the

Boys and then friends of friends. We were like an army. Mind you, that *was* a long time ago, almost when we were still Mods!

Jamie had played football for many years and, after he stopped playing, a number of former players formed a skittles team that plays in the city's 'clubs league'. He still plays once a week. Jamie is also an inveterate gambler. An opening remark in my research interview with him was that "if we weren't in lockdown, I'd be at the bookies right now, with my spending money". He elaborated that he operated on a weekly spending limit (he wouldn't say how much, but "it's quite a lot" and made a point to say that his wife has the same!) to indulge his twin vices of drinking and gambling: "I'm not a serious gambler but I can do what I like with my spending money; I worked hard for it all week, or all month I should say". Most Saturdays he leaves the house around 10:30, to buy a newspaper and spend £4.00 on the Lottery ("oh, there's another gamble: I get it on a Saturday, she gets it on a Wednesday"). He would then go to the bookies and often not get home until just before mid-day, on account of meeting and chatting to people on the way (and in the bookies). He bets on football as well as the horses, "because there's nothing better than watching a game if you've got a chance of winning something from it, it's more exciting, there's more of an edge". He waxed lyrical for some minutes over the detail of different stakes – "you can bet on the result, of course, but these days you can bet on first goal-scorer, or the minute of the first goal, almost anything" – and various forms of accumulator: "it's great when you win". Jamie looked askance when I told him that I had never been in a betting shop in my life!

When he's 'home' in Milltown (rather than working away, as he often is), Gary goes to the football with Spaceman and links up with the Boys, though – like Jamie – he readily admits to his 'bad habit' of gambling too much:

> I've always done it, H. I just love it. On the horses. I've always loved a flutter. I know it's a bad habit and I can easily do £50.00 a day. Not this online stuff. Down the bookies. Like I've always done. That's where I often see some of the other Boys.

Mack echoed Gary's remarks, stating that he often put a bit of money on the horses. He used to link up with the Boys in the bookies, but – unlike Gary – he increasingly uses online betting and, anyway, only stakes modest sums, usually "only about a fiver at a time". Other than that, he watches TV and YouTube videos: "yeah, I watch all the sport, you know, the football, snooker, darts, all of that". In contrast, his lifelong close friend Mark hardly ever watches television; as a postman, he goes to bed early (around 9 pm) and he doesn't have Sky – "it costs too much; I'm not paying that"!

One of the few surviving and thriving drinking holes in Milltown is the social club on the main road that divides the estate. Some of the Boys are stalwarts who, as young adults, became members (and, like Tommy, even members of the Committee) and – despite occasional bans – have never left, even if their attendance is not as frequent as it used to be: Jerry, Tommy, Mark, Denny and Mal could routinely be found 'up the club' rather than down the pub. But the social club is also used for symbolic occasions by virtually all of the other Boys. It was the venue for Marty's wake as well as where the Boys gathered after the funeral of Gary's son. Kelvin's wife held her 60th birthday party there. And I, too, held a party there in the early part of the Millennium to thank the Boys for their trust in me.

Unprompted, Tony concluded our discussion of his leisure time with the remark that it was "a long way from the West End", the social club in question. He could not have spoken a truer word, as he outlined the wide range of activities he pursues in his leisure time:

> Well, there's obviously the football at Anfield [Liverpool's ground], where I've got a season ticket. I don't go to every game. I pick and choose, and I go to finals. We're lucky enough to go on holiday. One of the good things about having your own business is that it gives you flexibility. I know some people with their own business work seven days a week. I get that, but normally I try to do just four days a week, so I have quite a lot of time off over the year. So, we've travelled a lot, mostly Europe, but we went to Alaska last year. That was nice. We've been to the States quite a few times, the Caribbean, stuff like that. Cruises, nice hotels.
>
> We like to eat out, so we do quite a few city-breaks where we go to nice restaurants. So, our leisure time is, yes, holidays, we like to go out to dinner, we like to go out with friends. We're very close to our daughters. Angie's [Tony's wife] a very good cook, so we like to eat well at home. I'm quite into wine, I like wine, I'm interested in wine. Something I might do more of when I've got a bit more time. Spanish. I like Spain. I went to night classes for four years to learn Spanish. I wouldn't mind taking that to the next level. So, yeah, in summary, that's about it.
>
> Oh, and I read, recently more the newspapers, rather than books. *The Times*, The *Sunday Times*, flick through *The i*, and occasionally, just to see what the enemy is doing, I will buy *The Guardian*. And I guess like most people I look at a lot of stuff online, on my phone. But I do like to pick up a physical newspaper on the weekend. There's so much in the Sunday papers. I suppose, like most men, I flick through the front page and then turn to the back pages, to the sport! And then I read some of the commentators. There are some I like a lot.

While Tony already has a diverse set of leisure interests, and some of the other Boys are fairly fixed in the ways in which they consume their leisure time, Kelvin talked at length about his dreams. He said he listened to 'a bit' of music (mainly old mod and ska tunes) and was one of the Boys who congregate in *The Vulcan* most Saturday nights and then go into town "though obviously lockdown has changed that at the moment". On the weekend in early July 2020 when I conducted my research interview with Kelvin, Tony had just been on the phone "rubbing it in that England was celebrating the pubs reopening". Kelvin has two vintage Vespa scooters (one 125 cc and the other 200 cc) that he wants to get back on the road:

> Yeah, there's loads of things I want to do, starting with building a workshop at the bottom of the garden in the new house, where I can work on the scooters, and other things …
>
> And I've always loved history. So, if I did retire [see Chapter 6] and had the money, I'd probably go travelling the world. I wouldn't just sit at home on my arse. I'd want to stay active. I'd do things I've always wanted to do. I'd go to Malaya [*sic*] because that's where my father was in the army. And I'd like to go to China, and Australia. I'm not really interested in the USA. I'd love to go to Jordan, to Petra, and to Peru, to Machu Picchu, to a place in Bolivia, those temples in Cambodia, India, the Taj Mahal. Stuff like that. The marvels of the world. I've been to the pyramids, but I'd love to go to the Valley of the Kings …

Yet while providing this long list of exotic destinations that he would like to see, Kelvin concluded with the rather more cautious remark that

> I don't think I've got any massive expectations left in life; I'd just like to see my kids doing well, which they are, and the world's got to be a better place for my grandkids, but you never know what's around the corner, so I never plan for what's around the corner, because you just never know. You never know.

of the Boys (neither of whom had ever been in serious trouble), he has a university degree.[67] Spaceman reflected on his lifetime association with the Boys:

> It's the funerals, I suppose, when you think about it most. And there's more and more of them. It's like the fucking Gambinos – everybody *always* turns up. You just *know* they're going to be there. I love *all* the Boys. Now you know that I haven't always got on with all of them, but I wouldn't judge any of them. Not all of them had the ball passed to them; they were on their own from the start. I don't hate any of them; just some fell off the cliff. I even cut myself off from the ones I knew best, like Tony and Jamie, and Dean and Gary. I didn't want them seeing me destroying myself through drinking. Mind you, Dean and I have been writing to each other – letters first, now email – since we both joined the Merchant Navy, since 1977. He's still in there, of course. Yes, still writing.
>
> I've done loads of drawing and paintings for Gary, including a picture of Adrian, that he's got on the wall.[68]
>
> It doesn't really matter if they understand what I'm on about or not. Some of them do – like Gordon, Dean or Kelvin; they're well read. Others, like Mark, and Ted, and Mack, well the conversation level is different. But I love them all. I love all the Boys. The Boys are honest with me. I trust them; I'd trust them with my life.

Spaceman talked further about fitting in with different individuals and sub-groups amongst the Boys. As he read novels and philosophy, he came across words he could not understand – "there were a couple of the Boys I'd ask, because they'd probably know, whereas if I asked Jamie [one of Spaceman's closest friends], you could give him fifty years and he still wouldn't know the answer".

At that very moment in the research interview, Spaceman's doorbell rang: it was none other than Jamie, delivering some food. Spaceman left his phone on the fence and I talked to Jamie, arranging a research interview with him in the process. Jamie is probably the most impressive and engaging comedian amongst the Boys:

> Care in the Community, Howard. Helping the elderly. Schweppes with quinine. Oh, and I've got some money out of the bank, for his drugs (only

---

67 Out of all the Boys, only Gordon and Spaceman contemplated post-16 education while they were at school (see *The Milltown Boys Revisited*, p.31 and p.39). Gordon pressed on, almost secretly, and went on to complete a BA degree in sociology. Spaceman was railroaded out of A level studies (Art and English) in the first term and left school to join the Merchant Navy, only returning to education in his late 30s and achieving a BA degree in fine art at the age of 42 (see *The Milltown Boys Revisited*, p.45 and p.87). Shaun also has a university degree, in electrical engineering, which he gained in his mid-30s (see footnote 58).

68 At Adrian's funeral, amongst the photographs projected, there was one of him playing with his cat. Spaceman has done a large oil painting of that moment, which hangs on the wall directly opposite the settee in Gary's living room.

kidding).Yesterday it was meals on wheels, Sunday lunch made by the good wife.Actually, it just gets me out of the house!

But Spaceman didn't see it like that at all. When he had retrieved his phone and Jamie had left, he insisted it proved the point:

I didn't ask him for help. He just turned up as soon as the lockdown was announced.We lived next door when we were **5 years old**!We were walking round the streets then; we're talking now. Fifty-five years ago....

The loyalty that surrounds the Boys is palpable. It exudes from every dimension of their relationships. In a telephone conversation with Tony, as he was driving home from work (from the distribution company where he is the co-owner) in a top-of-the-range Mercedes – such a far cry from the circumstances in which he grew up – he made the unsolicited observation that,

I still talk regularly to so many of the Boys. I've been away from Milltown for 35 years now but the reunions and relationships are magical... I don't know of anybody else – certainly not amongst the people I've got to know since then – who still have contact with such a number of people they've known since they were kids. I've known those boys since we were knee high to a grasshopper. It's a unique connection.

[12th May 2020]

In my research interview with Tony, he started by reporting that only the previous weekend he had spoken to Kelvin, Phil, Gary, Spaceman, had emailed Dean [who is still in the Merchant Navy], and had talked with Jamie only the day before – "you know, we talk a lot, we're still very close....Yeah, I must have spoken to Gary for at least an hour on Saturday, when I went for a walk". Tony said that Gary had been a 'great addition' to the catholic Boys, describing him as "a bit of an interloper who joined our gang". I did not ask directly about 'regrets', as I had in 2000, but Tony acknowledged that perhaps he had physically missed out on more events with the Boys than he would have wanted to:

If I had any regrets, well it's not really regrets, and it's not really pangs of guilt, but I have missed some of those bigger events – and I'm really talking about funerals, because parties are in the evening and on the weekend, so I've got to most of those, whereas funerals are in the daytime and in the week – so I've missed a few funerals and it's because it's been very difficult for me because of my business commitments, when my business partner's been away.

But, yes, I still get to as much as I can, even though I live quite a long way away. And the way I look at it... with the Boys. I look at all of those guys... and you know, if in life, I think that if you can count five really close friends on one hand, then I think you're a very lucky person and we're all much luckier than that, because I think we can count at least ten, just from the guys we grew up with.

Tony's viewpoint was corroborated in a different way but equally assertively by Jamie, who has lived in or on the doorstep of Milltown all his life:

> I'm a Milltown Boy through and through. I always used to go to the Home Guard with my dad, until he passed away. I'd meet the Boys every Sunday, for years, up *The Centurion*. I think you always go back to your roots. Although some traditions die out. It got harder to get up on Sunday after a Saturday night on the piss, and then you couldn't sit outside on the wall up *The Centurion* anymore, because they put those spikes on it. And then the pub shut down a few years ago. That put an end to that routine. But, as I've said, I still see the Boys in other ways.

The closure of so many of the pubs in Milltown has certainly curtailed regular contact between the Boys. Danny was once one of the regulars at *The Fountain*. You could *guarantee* finding him there most lunchtimes and early evening. Today, as noted earlier, *The Fountain* Boys have decamped to one of the social clubs or to *The Highbury*, where Paul is a regular. Danny says the pub always wants him to join its skittles team but he prefers to spend his time with his 'best mate', his grandson Alfie. Nevertheless, he drops into *The Highbury* after an increasingly rare round of golf on the municipal golf course, and he also sees some of the Boys at local rugby matches where their grandchildren are playing. Beyond that, contact with the Boys is generally limited to lengthy conversations during chance encounters in the street:

> One of the funniest things about the Boys I know best is that I wanted to fight a lot of them at first. Like Vic. Because he had a bit of a name, and I had a bit of a name, so you had to prove yourself. And you'd find some excuse for a fight, like 'what are you looking at?', and people would stand in the way, but sometimes things kicked off. Stan's first words to me were 'I'm going to fucking kill you', and I hadn't done nothing! And now we've been 'working' together for 29 years. He's my business partner! But because I had the name, he sort of targeted me. But then the police came. And after that we got on, and we've never looked back.
>
> And a lot of the other Boys, I've known since we were five or six, seven years of age. We were kids, playing football in the street and hanging around up the rec. The likes of Ted, Jerry – up the woods field for a kick around. Mack, Johnny, Richard, the Wilcox's, they were the ones in my street and then there were the other Boys who went up the rec, like Ryan and Trevor.
>
> We all grew up together as mates, doing things together, up the rec and by the shops. And I still see a lot of them. Even though not so much now because we haven't got *The Fountain* any more. But I'll go in *The Highbury* now and

again, after golf, and have a couple of pints and a little smoke with them, the ones who are there.

I don't really need them no more. I've got my family and they've got theirs. I like to see them, but if I don't see them, I don't see them. I can live without them. But when I do see them, we always stop and talk and it's always good to see them.

Having a 'name', as Danny put it, remains significant to this day. On one occasion when I visited Ted, as his health was declining, I spent a lot of the time talking on the doorstep with his 14-year-old son Brandon, who was very curious about what his father had been like at his age, particularly as Brandon has almost been excluded from school for his poor behaviour and Ted had told him that he should make the most of his schooling! Apparently, Brandon had asked his school to get a copy of *Five Years* but the school had not been prepared to pay £120.00 for the one copy available at the time on Amazon.[69] Brandon knew I was 'the one who writes the books' or, alternatively 'dad's posh friend'. I was standing by the back door but, within earshot of Ted, I told Brandon that his father had not gone to an ordinary secondary school but had been in a residential school for 'bad boys'; I had met him, as I had met Danny, when he was on weekend leave from that school. Brandon asked me if his father had been 'hard'. I said that might be an understatement; I told Brandon that he is described in another book as (to quote it precisely), "a big lad, who could handle himself [and who] would beat up anyone who grassed him up". Ted interjected from his cushioned chair in the living room: "what you've got to understand, son, is that reputation was everything; it was the only thing that counted.... It was the only thing that mattered".

Mark described the Boys as 'very special', even though he didn't see so many of them any more:

> Yeah, special, very special. I mean, Kat is the best mate ever; he was my best man. But then there's Jerry, and Matt and Mal and Mack. Although I don't see some of them, like Matt, so much anymore, when you *do* see each other, you know, it's great. We all still get on really well. It's a shame I don't see Pete no more, but then he's moved away. I mean, I saw Danny a couple of days ago and we had a good chat. And when I came out of hospital, I saw Mack, who's got a colostomy bag – he's had one for a long time – and he said he could tell me all I'll ever need to know about it! So yeah, the Boys are very special. They've got to be, Howard, haven't they; we've known each other since we were knee high to a grasshopper.[70] The trouble is that, with some of them

---

69 The original retail price of *Five Years* was £2.25 (with, in keeping with the post-punk culture at the time, a free badge if you bought a copy from me!). It has sometimes reached £100.00 + on Amazon, but when Brandon asked me about it, I went on Google and found a copy for him, on eBay for £9.99.

70 The very same expression that had been used by Tony.

at least, you never know where they are from one day to the next, like Matt. And not so many of them go up the club any more.

Matt, the only one of the Boys in my follow-up study with wholly BAME heritage (both his natural parents came from Barbados), and one of the few black kids amongst the Boys, talked about not feeling any sense of racism from the Boys themselves, though he said he was routinely called a 'black bastard' by many of their fathers. Matt said that this never particularly concerned him. The following quotation can only be understood with the knowledge that, because many gulleys round the side of houses were sometimes overgrown or blocked off (today they are securely fenced off[71]), one could only reach the back garden of many houses in Milltown, including my own, by going through the house:

> If one of the Boys was going to have a party in his back garden and I showed up, I'd often get 'I'm not having that black bastard in my house', so we'd just have the party in the front instead [laughs].

And he followed up this poignant note with the observation, "When you're around people who are like a family, you don't think of colour". Looking back, he said, it was now clear in his mind that he had often been 'picked out', including by the police, almost certainly on account of his skin colour, but he said he had hardly ever dwelt on that possibility at the time. He reminisced about meeting in a pub 20 years ago, with Mark, Spaceman, Jerry, Pete, Nutter and Nick, remarking not on their diversity but the bond of their shared roots.[72] Not that he sees many of them any more:

> If I see any of the Boys today, I still stop and talk to them. But it doesn't happen very often. There was a time, when I lived in Milltown, when they meant everything to me. Now I'm cut off, isolated, a bit of a hermit. But I still know they're there if I need them.

Mark's take on racism (or the lack of it) in Milltown was quite similar to that of Matt – people used the language but didn't really mean it – and indeed Mark included Matt in his recollections. These started, however, with a quite unsolicited set of observations about the *Black Lives Matter* street protests in June 2020 that followed the killing of George Floyd in the USA by a Minneapolis police officer, as the latter knelt on Floyd's neck for over eight minutes, even though he was crying

---

71 See footnote 34.

72 It was quite a remarkable gathering. Mark and Nutter were confirmed heavy drinkers; Spaceman was his unique, maverick self, drinking soft drinks as a recovering alcoholic; Nick, too, was teetotal at the time; Jerry joined us with Rachel, in her wheelchair; Pete lounged on a settee in extremely louche, camp style; and Matt was wearing a flamboyant Caribbean 'calypso' T-shirt. I was rather moved by the palpable camaraderie within such diversity.

out that he could not breathe. He had been arrested for supposedly trying to pay for groceries with a counterfeit $20 bill:

> It's absolutely disgusting what happened to him… but look at all these people now, jumping on the pissing bandwagon. You know, two weeks ago, none of these would have given that man a 20-dollar bill. Half of them at least are hypocrites. You know, I wish we could go back to when we were growing up. Well, this lot are going on about slaves and those statues; well, when we younger, we were all allowed out all the time and we could do whatever we liked, but the likes of Matt and the other black kids, well they had to stay in and do the housework, peel the spuds and gut the fish… you know, they were treated like slaves in their own houses! They were not allowed outside until they'd done all that. It was the same with Kat. The younger ones were the downtrodden because the older you were, the more bossy you were, and the less you had to do. And they're all going on about racism and racist language. Well, you know yourself, we used to call each other everything, didn't we? I'm not saying we should go back to those dark days, but they wasn't dark days to us, Howard. Because even the coloured people, we were all the same, we'd call *each other* all the names under the sun. You know, and I think where have we gone so far back that the black people feel so oppressed. You know, I just can't get my head round it.
>
> I did see it, mind, when we went to Sunderland,[73] to a friend's kid's christening, and we were walking along and across the road was Matt. Oh, and it was terrible up there, How, it was like going back 30 years, and this car went speeding past shouting out that they were going to run him over, at Matt. They looked at him gone off, up there. And, later, I was up at the bar in this pub, and I don't think they thought I was with him, 'cos these boys were talking, calling him all these things, and I said to them to go and say it to his face. Because, you know as well, Matt could handle himself if he needed to. I said to this bloke and his mates, 'go on, go and say it to his face, and I can tell you now, if you do, he'll lick the floor with all of you'. On his own, without anyone else. And they just walked out the pub, still mumbling things about Matt under their breath. So bigoted.
>
> Just so bigoted. You never saw that down here. But when you went up there, where there are hardly any blacks, it was like stepping back in time. They were just so fucking racist and you could see they meant it, because they'd obviously never had that much to do with coloured people.

---

73 The north-east of England has become something of a weather-vane for the shifting political allegiances of the British white working-class, particularly in the decision, in 2016, by the UK to leave the European Union and, in 2019, the election of the Conservative government with a significant majority. Immigration, and party-political attitudes to immigration has been one, though by no means the only factor. For a very interesting analysis and reflection of these issues specifically in relation to Sunderland, see Hayman (2017).

Mark continued to argue that, although he had grown up at a time of explicitly racist TV programmes such as *Till Death Us Do Part*[74] and *Love Thy Neighbour*, there had never been any real animosity towards black people in Milltown and that everybody had got on well together: "today, you can't say anything out of place, for fear of causing offence. It's just gone OTT". He concluded his thoughts by referring, once again, to the killing of George Floyd: "by the way, How, they should do all four of those policemen, they should throw the fucking book at them".

Vic, with mixed race origins (his father from Nigeria, his mother from Ireland), had a very different view about racism in Milltown. He generally agreed with Mark and Matt that a great deal was just 'routine' language without malicious intent, but he also spoke at length about how he actively avoided those he had perceived as 'really' racist rather than those who "just used the words". I had reminded him that he once remarked that he had only really realised he was black when he went to prison:

> I mean, you come from an area where there is black and white everywhere and then you go to a place where everybody is separated. My idea of getting on was the black and the white all together, but when I went inside, it was either with the blacks or the whites. If I wasn't with the blacks or the whites I had to be on my own, so that's the thing I didn't like. Because the whites didn't want me. So it made me feel more black. I *had* to be more black. It had never bothered me before. I never thought about it until I went to those places. I'd never been called names before, you know, like nigger. There it was in your face.
>
> *(The Milltown Boys Revisited, p. 94)*

With remarkable consistency in his recollections and perspectives and a tinge of sadness, which pervades Vic's commentary on many of his experiences throughout his life, he responded to my reminder as follows:

> You know me, I don't distinguish black or white, me.... I get it [racial abuse] from black people and I get it from white people, 'cos I'm mixed race. I get it from both fucking sides! Most people only get it from one side! But I don't take too much notice any more not now that I'm older. No, I just look at people and smile; sometimes I even say 'yes, I am, you're right, I am a black bastard, and if you really want to see a black bastard, I can behave like one'.... That's usually shut them up, because of my size.[75]

74 The central character was Alf Garnett, a bigoted, reactionary white working-class man. The creator of the series claimed to have written the series to challenge racism, but it was subjected to criticism that those who watched it tended to support Garnett's racist views.

75 Vic was talking to me just before the *Black Lives Matter* street protests that followed the killing of six-foot-six George Floyd by a white police officer, in Minneapolis in the USA. In one of Floyd's obituaries, it was noted, "But he, Big Floyd, was famous mostly for his size – a size that made people think he was not gentle or calm, but a fighting person" ('The life pressed out', *The Economist*, 6 June

> You know, How, growing up in an area like Milltown, I never really experienced really bad racism. It was just there, it was there and it was an everyday thing, 'cos most of my friends were white anyway and then, when I did go to prison [in fact, a senior Detention Centre], and the officers were using them terms … well, I'd be known as the black sheep of the family, because I was from fucking Wales, with all its sheep, ha ha, and the other language they used towards me there, it was horrible, it was fucking horrible. And there was nothing you could do about it. You just had to stand there and take it. It was horrible.

The paradox in Vic's perspectives is that while he is relatively accepting of supposedly innocuous racist remarks coming from all-white individuals (though not from those whose comments he understands to be malicious), he is completely intolerant when they emanate from those who themselves are mixed race. His own son fought back after racial abuse from somebody of Maltese origin; Jake was subsequently charged with assault. Vic had gone to court with him, to discover that the father of the 'victim' was an old acquaintance from Milltown. Charges were, as a result, not pressed and the case was dropped, but Vic has never spoken to the father since:

> and I see him in Milltown, and I still won't speak to him now, and that must have been twenty years ago. It makes me sick, because he must never have told his kids that they're mixed race too, the same as my son. I'd said to him in the court, there must be something wrong with you – your own fucking children don't know what they *are*. You should be installing [*sic*] that in your children, make them proud of what they are, whatever it is, whether it's mixed race, white, black, fucking pink or blue. I've never ever hassled my son for beating someone up when it's about that. If somebody wants to call you a black bastard, you treat 'em like one, be a black bastard back to them. Be horrible, let 'em see how it makes you feel. Because it makes you feel like fucking shit.…

He was particularly scathing about one particular individual who had recurrently racially insulted him in his childhood, despite his own part-Arab ethnic origins:

> That man, going all the way back to school, he used to stand on the wall and call me all the black B's under the sun, and I used to go home and tell my grandmother and she said, when you go out on the street and he calls you them names again, tell him to look at his father. And we were by the garages

---

2020, p.82). Much the same applied to Vic. The 'labelling theory' originated by Lemert (1951) and developed by Becker (1963) would fit very well with Vic, as would the idiom 'give a dog a bad name', which has been defined as "said when someone has been accused of behaving badly in the past, with the result that people expect them to behave like that in the future" (Cambridge Dictionary).

and he was giving it to me again and who should come out of his house but his father, Assam, and he gave his boy a slap for calling me names, but Stan's always been like that – he always thought he was white. I don't know why, but he's always gone on about the fucking darkies. For some reason he wants to be whiter than white. I've never wanted to have anything to do with that man.

Given that Stan[76] is mates, indeed very close mates, with some of the other Boys, as well as being Danny's 'business partner', this has driven something of a wedge into the contact Vic has had with them; indeed, it has pushed Vic further away, to the point where Vic now connects almost exclusively with Ted, who lives some distance from Milltown. During the Covid-19 lockdown, Vic – who had been living in Milltown in the house of a relative – decamped to Ted's house, hoping he may soon be allocated a place to live nearby.

Yet Vic remains strikingly loyal to his old 'muckers', as he calls them. He had once turned up one day in *The Fountain* – which exuded a very intimidating ambience to somebody unfamiliar with it and not known to its regulars (who comprised mainly individuals, not necessarily all from Milltown, involved in illicit activities of one kind or another)[77] – to discover that Pete, as camp as a camp gay man can be, had been in, looking for him. Vic was immediately 'looking out for him', leaping to his defence:

> Pete was always one of my top mates. I remember going in *The Fountain* one day and it was 'oh, there was this fucking queer fellow come in, looking for you'. And I said 'who?'. And somebody said it was Pete. And they made some comments about him. So I said 'you'd better not have been giving him any crap, because if I find out you have, I'll fucking fill you in… he was my fucking school mate'. That's the way I am, anyway – don't give some fella a hard time because of his sexuality. And I'm certainly not going to have it from anyone, if they do that with someone who's my mate.

There has *always* been a remarkable sense of loyalty amongst the Boys but perhaps Vic expresses it more powerfully on account of his own deeply-felt experience of racism, about which he has become increasingly conscious as he has grown older.

Some of the Boys are more cut off, but there are still often impressive levels of contact between many of them. Paul says he rarely goes out of his way to communicate with most of the others but "when I see them, I always stop and have a chat with them":

---

76 Bizarrely, as I was writing this up, on 21 May 2020, Stan sent me a Facebook friends request. I had not seen him for years, but obviously we share some mutual 'friends'. I did not accept it.

77 It was often likened to *The Slaughtered Lamb*, the pub where two walkers sought shelter in the film *American Werewolf in London*; full of strange and mean looking local people, the pub went silent when the two Americans walked in.

But, like I says, everyone's got their own lives these days. They're all doing other things. Sometimes some of the Boys come to the pub and then I talk to them but I don't really go looking for them. But if they come to the pub, then we'll have a pint together. I'm drinking with a different crew these days, like in their late 60s, 70s – I like listening to their crap, hear them talking their shit! I love it. That's what I does. Sorry to go on. That's my life now.

Kelvin, who told me that he "wasn't very good with words", articulated the closeness of the Boys more graphically than many of the others:

Yeah, we're all still pretty close. Of course, we have our ups and downs. We still have our arguments, our bickerings. But we've had a strong friendship over the years and it's been a long friendship. I think we're a group of guys who, if one of us was in trouble, we'd move the earth to help out. You know, if we could do it, we would do it. We're lucky to know each other.

Yeah, if you look at us, I mean, not just the catholic boys but also the likes of Jerry, Pete, Gary as well as Spaceman and Jamie – *all* those kind of guys that we've known through all these years. I mean, we all had different traits and when you think of that it's surprising that we all got on so well, 'cos we all had different interests and we all had different views, but the one thing we did have in common was our friendship. We were all comfortable with each other. We didn't hide anything from each other – well, family life, we didn't tend to talk about – and we all said it how it was. We were all close. We all looked after each other, watched out for each other. We were like a family, I suppose, really, you know what I mean. We were just lucky to be such good mates. We were lucky to have each other.

I mean, some of us have known each other for 55 years. I've known all the Boys since we were 4/5 years old. Some of them from birth, 'cos Spaceman's mother and my mother went to school together, Martin's [not one of the Boys in my study] mother went to school with my mother – and we all grew up in prams together, before we even went to school!

Whether it is choice or fate, as Spaceman put it, when reflecting on the Boys and their strikingly different pathways in life, they were bound together by three key things – their shared roots, their mutuality through good times and bad, and their *music*. They were not all fans of the same artists or even the same genres of music, though there was an almost ubiquitous love of Bowie. But Spaceman noted that if you named certain songs they immediately evoked either individuals or moments in their lives:

We've got a million shared memories. There's a song for everyone and everything – soundtracks of connection. You just picture the Boys in different places. Play *Five Years* and I think immediately of Marty or Ted. *Mr Know-It-all* by Stevie Wonder, and you'd think of Gary. *All the Young Dudes* by Mott the

Hoople, you'd think of Denny. *Get Down and Get With It* by Slade – and you think of Tommy. And so it goes on… Roxy Music, The Clash. All that punk and glam rock. *Una Paloma Blanca* by Jonathan King – and you think of the Boys sniffing glue over the woods.[78] Even Dylan, and you think of Alex (even if that was probably because of you). And these days, we just think of *When I'm Sixty-Four* and hope we get that far!

The musical associations spread not only far and wide but also some way back. Jerry was invariably linked to his favourite singer: Elvis Presley!

---

78 A very surprising 'soundtrack of connection'? *Una Paloma Blanca* was a massive hit for Jonathan King in 1975. For some unknown reason, the Boys rewrote the words in their minds and when they were in the woods getting high on glue they would start to sing it at the top of their voices: 'We are the glue-bag sniffers, we sniff it all of the day, we are the glue-bag sniffers, no-one will take…. Our glue-bags away' (see *Five Years*, p.28).

13

IDENTITY AND SELF-IMAGE

"We know how to get by... we always have"

(Kelvin)

"We're from Milltown, we don't cry"

(Spaceman)

"I'm a Rec-Boy through and through"

(Paul)

It is fascinating to hear the Boys talk amongst themselves. It can be hard to believe they are 60. They talk with all the bravado and gusto of teenagers, rarely conceding their age or sometimes failing health. They recurrently bemoan the 'cotton wool kids' of today, recalling that they were brought up 'tough', usually in large families and certainly on a 'hard' council estate, where they had learned to survive from an early age. Most significantly, they had learned "not to back down". Just occasionally now, however, they admit to doing so, even if it is "not in our nature". They reported moments when they encountered the "cheeky little fuckers today, lippy bastards" in the street and opted for the quiet life: "otherwise they'll be all over you like a pack of hyenas". One on one, they usually maintained, there would be no problem and no contest: "I may not be as fast or as strong as I once was, but I could still take them out". For those who had dealt with brutal fathers, violent older brothers, abusive staff in children's homes, sadistic and racist prison officers and what the Boys called the MUFTI (the hit squad who came for those who 'thought they were something' when in custody), they had every reason to believe that they could still hold their own with the young upstarts of today, some of whom are, of course, they concede reluctantly but simultaneously with a modicum of pride, their own children and, as the years have passed, grandchildren.

Matt, during his reflection on his life course and the undulation between the exhilarating heights of failed criminality (which would have brought very long custodial sentences, had he been caught) and the humiliating depths of low-level employment (out of which he still managed to salvage some sense of dignity and status, notably in his persona as the 'Glass Man' – see Chapter 6), made the following telling observation:

> I'm too crazy for my own good. I never found the balance in my life. I'm a peaceful man at heart. I don't want to trouble anyone and I don't want no trouble from anyone. Do you see what I'm saying, How? But I know I bully the bullies. I want to bully the bullies. And that includes the police. That's stopped me in my tracks so many times. Just when I thought things were working out. I think I've always been looking for that pot of gold at the end of the rainbow and now I've just got to accept I've not been looking right!

Having brushed with death, for different reasons, on more than one occasion, and now afflicted, since the operation on his brain, with what he described as 'working memory loss' (he said he would not even remember me interviewing him, though he could remember life some time ago), Matt said he did not really know the 'new Matt'. With his new medication, he was calmer now, but all he really had left were his memories.

The strange thing about the Boys is how their powerful shared collective identity is simultaneously a parasol for their pronounced individuality, even amongst some of the sub-groupings of the Boys who shared even more identical origins. I noted in *The Milltown Boys Revisited* (p.189) that Tony remains unconditionally loyal to Spaceman, though he has ascended to the heights of middle-class respectability, while, at least for a while, Spaceman plummeted to the depths of crime and drug addiction. Here is Spaceman in 2020:

> I've never made comparisons with any of the others. If I did, I would hurt them and I'd hurt myself. Look at fucking five-star Beechy [Tony]. He's so fucking rich. He always wanted to better himself, you know, go from egg on toast to veal cutlets. I had different dreams. All I ever wanted to be was an artist, although I forgot about it for about twenty years! I've never felt sorry for myself. I'm proud of myself. I suppose when I got my degree, I was really positive, direct, focused. I just wanted an ordinary job, so I could paint the rest of the time. I didn't know that my health would get in the way. And I definitely didn't know my degree would get in the way, a bit like my Milltown address did before! You can't get a normal job if you've got a degree! But I've been selling my paintings, which is something Van Gogh never did in his lifetime…

Spaceman admitted he was something of a 'chameleon', adapting in order to fit in with different crowds. He reminded me he had had to do that since he was a child – you did not want to admit to reading Camus or Sartre to a mate who only read football magazines. He said that his opportunities to mix with different groups throughout his life had given him the opportunity for "reflection and revelation, a process of discovery about who I am"; after all, how many people have been both a prisoner and a student, *not* at the same time?

As far as Spaceman was concerned, Ted "had had it tougher, even tougher than the rest of us; he never really had a chance". Spaceman's view was that Ted's domineering identity had been forged through the imperative to survive; losing his parents when he was a child and then being shunted across the country to a sequence of child care institutions, and the brutalising experiences that they had engendered, had made him "even harder than the rest of us".

Gary was arguably more critical, yet ultimately not judgemental about any of the Boys, even though he was forthright in defining some of them in a different way. He had always maintained that *he* had done well because he had inherited a strong work ethic from his father, who had also been a painter and decorator. At the age of 60, Gary proudly noted he had been doing that work for more than 30 years: "you make your own luck", he said. He conceded, however, that it might have been very different. In *The Milltown Boys Revisited* (pp.74–75), Gary recalls his delinquent teenage years and the moment he "knew it was time to stop". I wrote that "He immersed himself in work and has never been in any trouble since". But Gary continues to acknowledge that he, too, could have ended up like many of *The Fountain* Boys:

> H, I grew up with those Boys. The difference was that they didn't want to work. They never planned to work. I started off, as you know, on one of those schemes and fiddling the dole, drinking at lunchtime. I enjoyed it. I could've easily jumped on that side. I was an inch away. I'd been up for affray once and I was up for it again, after another fight. My barrister got me off. I got found Not Guilty. But he said to me, 'do you realise how serious the charge was?' He said I would've gone to prison. That's when things really sunk in. I had to change my ways. I wanted to earn money and I had to do it legally.
>
> Those other Boys, they've all ended up in prison. And they've done a lot of time, a lot of time. We're talking 10, 20, even 25 years in all. All those years. So, so sad. And they've never had a job. Some of them are still on the dole and on the golf course. But most of them can't get up in the morning; a lot of them are suffering from ill-health and paranoia. They say they're happy, and they seem happy, but I'm not so sure. But, H, I'm still comfortable with them. We still get on. They're bad boys. I'm not. But there's mutual respect. We go back a long, long way.
>
> If you want to make something of yourself in this world, you've got to put the hours in. People are proud of me and what I've achieved. I'm proud of me, H! I've done well.

The collective heritage of the Boys really does cover elements of striking individuality, as Kelvin tried to explain. He, along with Mark and a number of the other

Boys (some featured in this book, some not, but all known to me) have classically gone on holiday together, year after year, organised by one of the Boys' wives. This arrangement has continued throughout their lives, even after their children have grown up. And yet one year he had not gone with the group, electing instead to spend the money on a scooter. In discussing his imminent house move, he explained that one major dilemma would be where to put all his clothes – three wardrobes full! I had often commented, over the years, on his 'sartorial elegance', where he nearly always stood out in the crowd, particularly in the days when he was a 'Mod':

You see, How, you've got to understand some of the differences amongst us. Yes, I've got *so many clothes*. Some of the Boys just aren't so bothered about things like that. But I've got so many clothes, it's unbelievable. It's absolutely ridiculous. I just love my clothes. I like to look smart when I go out. And a lot of that comes from when I was younger. When I was growing up I can never, ever remember being hungry, you know, going to bed feeling hungry, like some of the Boys, but I never had much in the way of clothes. I do remember my mum and dad giving us everything they could, but I always remember being a bit late with the fashion, because they could only get me stuff when they had the money. So, when all the Boys were wearing brogues, then only four or five months down the line I'd get a pair, only to find the Boys were wearing loafers. You know, the fashion changed so quick. I'd come out, saying 'hey look at my new brogues' and they'd go 'oh yeah, OK'…. You get me? I was always behind.

And I think, because of that, I've always had this thing in my head that, if I can, I've got to have it *now*. I've got to be *ahead*. Since I've been able to pay for things myself, I've always got what I wanted, my wife has had what she wanted and my kids have had what they wanted. If there was money in the house. When times were good. Don't get me wrong, there have been some hard times, when I didn't indulge, but not so many, so if the kids wanted something, they'd have it.

And I've always looked tidy and smart – and I got it *first*! Which I know sounds a bit selfish. But I've always had this thing about being ahead of the game with style. And so I've got loads of clothes, far too many clothes, but I know that never, ever, when I go out with the Boys, can they say that I look scruffy or my stuff is too out of date. It's crazy. But I think it was also the reason that some of the Boys used to steal, back in the day, because they wanted the latest fashion and they wanted it *now* – not like when I got it, when things had moved on!

This is all so reminiscent of the words in Danny's *Rec-Boy* song, where he talks about 'takes cash and the fags' in order to get 'on a par' with others, even if that often meant going 'too far'. At the university, Spaceman conveys to my students the abject poverty experienced by many of the Boys – meagre meals (it is noticeable how some of the Boys make the pointed remark that at least they always had food on the table), hand-me-down clothing, shoes with holes in them plugged with newspaper, and significant physical brutality in family life. It was not uncommon for *me* to hear from the Boys, in the early days I knew them, of having been locked in cupboards overnight, or whipped with a leather belt as a punishment for transgressing what were often very variable and inconsistent domestic rules, though they rarely told each other of these episodes and experiences. Literally, they suffered in silence. The Boys' fathers inhabited cultures of aggressive masculinity (see Connell 1995). If they worked at all, they were usually involved in tough, physical, dirty work. They usually sought refuge and respite from the brutalities of their own daily working lives by socialising and drinking heavily down the pub, and then – after staggering home – they would visit the same brutalities on their wives and children. Some of the Boys used to tell me of the sheer terror they felt about going home at night, hoping that their fathers would not hear them come in, or that they would be asleep before their fathers came in and, if their fathers were going to vent their anger on somebody in the house, it would not be them. It was not, of course, always brutal. When parents (essentially, though not always, fathers) were sober and not stressed on account of work or lack of income, they had indulged the Boys, sometimes with money and sometimes with attention. But much of the time it was not like that.

No wonder the Boys sought to establish a more meaningful profile in public. In *Five Years* (p.16) I wrote about 'ostentatious smoking' around the age of 11, standing near the bus stop and blowing smoke rings, inviting admonishment from those alighting the bus that 'you're too young to be doing that'. For the Boys, smoking was a symbol of their autonomy, independence and maturity. If they hadn't stolen cigarettes from opportunist theft, robbing houses or parents' packets, they were assisted by the local shopkeeper who was willing to sell them 'separates'[79] (one cigarette at a time, which was strictly illegal).

Smoking was but one facet of an image the Boys sought to project from an early age. That image – the Doc Martin ox blood boots (or, as Kelvin noted, the brogues or loafers), the Lee jeans, the Ben Sherman shirts, the Wrangler denim jacket, and so much more – cost money and was in constant flux. The Boys did their best to acquire the resources to keep up, from spotting the moment when family might provide a handout to shoplifting, burglary and theft. In that way, most of them kept up and many remain preoccupied with 'style', one way or another, to this day.

79 Milltown experienced some violent riots in the early 1990s. There were many media and academic explanations for them, from racism to the breach of old agreements as to which shops were allowed to sell what. My take, derived from what the Boys told me, was that an Asian family that had taken over the general store was resented because they were not willing to sell 'separates' (individual cigarettes), split packets of biscuits in two and sell just half (at a mark-up, of course), or advance small amounts of credit ahead of dole day Thursday. The previous shopkeeper had made a fortune doing these things and was much loved because he did so. Local people took it for granted as custom and practice, and took umbrage when the new owners did not follow suit. A brick through the window triggered the riots. See Campbell (1993).

PART III

12

CLOSER THAN FAMILY

Talking about camaraderie, when we were all in Tenerife, me, Tommy, Tommy's kid brother Chris, Mal, and we got talking to this old couple and we told them we was all mates from schooldays, from the same small area and they just couldn't get over it. The man said, 'what, you've been mates all this time, and here you are, still together, and you've all come on holiday together?'. He said, 'well I can't believe that, I can't get over that'. He said he didn't see any of his schoolmates no more. He looked at us and he said 'That's just fantastic, unbelievable'. He seemed completely taken aback by it. Basically, if we can get the flights and we can get the same time off work, then we still all go together. We always have.

(Mark)

One question I asked of all the Boys was, having gone such very different ways through the life course, how much they still felt connected to those beyond their immediate circle of friends (such as Ted, Vic and Danny; the 'catholic' Boys; or the 'social club' Boys) – in other words, 'the Boys' as I had defined them, with their common geographical roots at the top of the estate.

Spaceman, though closely linked to the 'catholic' Boys (particularly Tony, Jamie and Gary), was, at the same time, something of an outlier in many respects. Like many of *The Fountain* Boys, he had been a shoplifter, alcoholic and drug taker, and like many of the 'catholic' Boys, he had had a secondary school education that produced some basic qualifications and was more into punk than rock; his wild and reckless behaviour was more extreme than the others. The style of 'Revisited' on the cover of the last book is more than a nod to the cover of The Sex Pistols' *Never Mind the Bollocks*. Like a third of the Boys featured in *The Milltown Boys Revisited*, Spaceman had experienced imprisonment as an adult; along with just two others

14

LOOKING BACK

In 2000, I asked the Boys both to look back on their lives and to look forward to what they felt was in store for them in the future.[80] I had no thought at the time that I might be writing about them again another 20 years later. This time, however, though I have occasionally covered them looking back throughout this text, this section is *my* reflection on a lifetime of contact with and research on the Milltown Boys. I do not anticipate writing about them again – 'The Milltown Boys at 80' – though you never know!

The Milltown Boys were *never* a gang. University courses that have made use of my previous writing about them have often endeavoured to depict them in that way but even cursory scrutiny would reveal that they possessed few of the core criteria within any of the diverse and contested criminological definitions of a gang. They were a large group of individuals, positioned and socialised within multiple and overlapping sub-groups, whose predominant shared characteristic was that they had all grown up within a stone's throw of each other, in an area of pronounced socio-economic deprivation. Indeed, even by the general 'working-class' standards of Milltown, the streets where most of the Boys grew up were, on many indicators from Census data, disproportionately deprived. That small mosaic of roads, avenues, 'closes' and cul-de-sacs was identified in a community study some years later, through a considered analysis of key Census data such as levels of unemployment and no-car households, as the 'critical patch' for social intervention (see Williamson

---

80 This was the hardest part of those interviews. As I have noted again in this book, the Boys are reluctant to look too far back or too far forward. It can be painful, and risky – they prefer not to think about it. When I asked about 'regrets', they tended to deflect the question through launching into either Frank Sinatra's or Sid Vicious' version of *My Way* (usually the latter!): 'regrets, I've had a few …' There is a pervasive sense of 'what's done, is done' and 'qué sera, sera' (see *The Milltown Boys Revisited*, pp.211–234, and pp.35–36).

and Weatherspoon 1985). On the home-made Monopoly board that the Boys and I made together in the 1970s, these streets were the brown and blue ones at the bottom of the board – from 'Old Kent Road' to 'Pentonville Road'. To set that in perspective, the street where I lived – in a two-bedroom, one-living room middle terrace house in a cul-de-sac on the edge of the 'critical patch' – was judged by the Boys to be equivalent to 'Vine Street', about half way round the board. I lived in the north of the estate but not 'up the top', where most of the Boys came from.

The title of Laub and Sampson's (2003) book *Shared Beginnings, Divergent Lives* could not be more apposite in also capturing the story of the Milltown Boys. For them too, what had been very solidly shared beginnings led to phenomenally divergent lives. That was evident even by the age of 18; it was what I was already writing about in *Five Years*. Despite the overlaps, which persisted into adult life, various sub-groups amongst the Boys had already solidified by their early 20s. Some (like Tony, Shaun and Gordon and especially Pete) had broken away, in many respects, almost completely – geographically, occupationally, domestically and, to some extent, culturally. Some (like Jamie, Spaceman, Kelvin, Jerry and Derek) took a bit longer to 'go missing', as the Boys sometimes put it. Others (like Danny, Denny, Mark, Mack, Paul, Nathan, Trevor, Ryan and Tommy) never went missing; they are still 'names' on the estate. But, with one or two exceptions (notably Pete and Shaun), all the Boys retained some level of attachment to Milltown or at least to the peer group of their childhood and youth.

I grew up alongside young people in the care system. My father was a child care officer (social worker) and he frequently took me with him on visits to children's homes, assessment centres, remand homes and approved schools. Through those experiences I met many individuals who were uncannily like the Milltown Boys, though of course I did not know that at the time. They prepared me well for what was to come. I had to adjust to their world, which was not easy for a boy who spoke with a middle-class accent, went to a direct grant school and was often dressed in a 'posh' school uniform. Just as Paul might as well have had THIEF written on his forehead, so I might as well have had SWOT or POSH written on mine. On the surface, I had nothing in common with those kids. But I was willing to learn, in particular absorbing their musical preferences. Harold Melvin and The Blue Notes, The Supremes and The Temptations were a long way from my peer group's interest in Led Zeppelin, Black Sabbath and Jimi Hendrix, or Bob Dylan, Simon and Garfunkel, and Fairport Convention. And though I went to an exclusively rugby-playing school, I preferred football and I was a pretty good player. The kids in the cottage homes wanted me on their side.

I was also a kind of 'youth worker' from an early age,[81] first establishing a youth club in the new community centre in my own village, and subsequently helping out at a nearby church youth club. I was an early member of 'Young Oxfam', a

---

81 See Williamson, H. (2017), 'Winning Space, building bridges – What youth work is all about', in H. Schild *et al.*, *Thinking Seriously About Youth Work*, Strasbourg: Council of Europe and European Commission

rapidly-growing youth organisation in the 1960s, raising money through various events and later, beyond the charity, campaigning for greater political commitment to overseas aid. I volunteered on Family Service Unit summer camps for 'deprived children'. I helped to build an adventure playground in Balsall Health in Birmingham[82]. In many of these settings, I came across children and young people who bore more than a passing resemblance to some of the Milltown Boys. In short, I was more or less 'ready' for the Boys when, eventually, I came upon them. This had nothing to do with any academic fieldwork skills and everything to do with a side of my upbringing the significance of which, until I arrived in Milltown, I had hardly acknowledged.

So, when the young Marty asked me to lend him a 'tenner' outside a budget supermarket in Milltown, shortly after I had moved there (see *The Milltown Boys Revisited*, p.3), I took it in my stride, feeling neither intimidated nor keen to run. Rather, I was curious, and the exchange that followed paved the way for the study that ensued.

But it was always so much more than a study. I lived in Milltown for almost six years. I drank in the local pub. I played for the local football teams. It was not diffi-cult to strike up a relationship with 'the Boys', even though those I came to study were around six years younger than me. Today, that relationship would almost cer-tainly be considered rather strange. Indeed, it might well be viewed as suspicious. But everything was in public view. The Boys hung around the streets; I was often seen hanging about with them. There was an age mix that stretched almost to my more advanced years (another of the 'gatekeepers'[83] to the Boys, as Marty had been, was just a couple of years younger than me). And I am sure that had I behaved 'oddly', an older brother or parent would have been round to sort me out, warn me off, or worse.

Instead, relatively quickly, I was made very welcome in Milltown. I was considered something of a curiosity (I still am, by some) and many people never really understood what I did, apart from it being 'something at the university'. Initially, I was viewed as a 'sort of youth worker', which is exactly what I was when the Boys first knew me. Having learned from Marty that they spent a lot of time 'up

---

82 In the sixth form at school we were encouraged to do something for 'our poorer neighbours on our doorstep'. I volunteered with Care for the Elderly in Balsall Heath, visiting an elderly lady (Mrs Dixon) every Friday afternoon. Balsall Heath was a notorious red light, deprived area of Birmingham. Walking back from Mrs Dixon's Victorian terraced house one day, I turned the corner to find students unloading railway sleepers on to some waste ground. I offered to help and continued to do so for a number of Fridays after that. This was the foundation of the St. Paul's Adventure Playground that grew to become the well-known St. Paul's Community Project, run by Dr Dick Atkinson (see Atkinson 1995).

83 Successful participant observation studies invariably depend on the outsider (researcher) having a 'gatekeeper' to let them in and vouch for them. The classic example is William Foote Whyte's 'Doc' (Whyte 1943). Doc was a central and critical figure within the group Whyte studied. That is not always the case. Researchers have to be attuned to the possibility that the individual who steps for-ward to 'take care' of them may be a marginal and less than influential figure in the group they are hoping to study!

the Rec', I ventured up there to discover the 'adventure playground' that doubled as a rather downbeat youth club; it was an old school building on the edge of the recreation ground. I quickly found myself volunteering at the 'club'. I was a second-year undergraduate student, with no thoughts in my head to pursue postgraduate studies. I thought I was going to be a social worker. Only when the opportunity presented to do a PhD did I start to discuss being a 'researcher' with the Boys and to describe myself as a university researcher to others. Even though this was true, it was not always considered plausible to everyone I knew. Some of the older people down the pub thought it might be a ruse and that in fact I was on the dole. After all, I seemed to be around a lot in the day. Every story in Milltown was open to interpretation! You never quite knew what was the truth. As Danny prefaced my interview with him in 2000, "it's going to be hard to tell the truth to you because I've spent my life lying – either to the police or down the social".

Irrespective of what people really knew about me, I was made welcome. Marty's grandmother would invite me round for Sunday lunch, with Marty, his brother and her boyfriend. We used to sit on the settee in a row, eating it in front of the TV. Jerry's father always asked me in to have a glass of whisky every Christmas. Shopkeepers got to know me. I was known in all the pubs. And ending up playing for three of Milltown's soccer teams (and captaining two of them) did me no harm in terms of embedding myself within other parts of community. As a result of all these activities, I became closely entwined in Milltown's social fabric, known not only to the Boys I was studying but to their brothers and sisters and wider families. I became a 'name' in a rather different way.

I had learned as an undergraduate about the 'norm of reciprocity' (see Chapter 3). In my final year of undergraduate studies, when I was already living in Milltown, I went to listen to Howard Parker speak about his own very recently-published participant observation study of car radio thieves in Liverpool (Parker 1974), one of the catalysts for my own study. In the pub after his talk, I was curious to find out what had become of the 'Roundhouse boys'. Parker said he didn't know. I was bemused. He told me he had lost touch. The boys apparently resented him because he had written a book about them and they presumed (quite wrongly) that he was now a wealthy author, "like Harold Robbins", Parker said. The Roundhouse boys thought he had 'used' them. Parker said he couldn't go back.

This story stayed with me and, when I started the 'study' of the Milltown Boys, I determined to make sure that, when asked and if possible, I would try to give something back. Initially, I was given credit for going to court with the Boys: it may have been a core part of my research activity, but the Boys and their parents were very appreciative of it; they saw it as me keeping them company and proving support. In 2000, I was rather shocked when, as Mal's wife opened the door and I introduced myself, she hugged me. I had never met her before, but she told me that she knew I'd been to Bristol with Mal as a kid, when he was in court for an offence of football violence: "he's told me all about it so many times, so I feel I know you already".

Beyond things that were interpreted as 'help' when they were in fact part of my research, I spent a lot of time helping people to understand and complete forms and applications – it took me by surprise that so many people were not literate. But it gave me the opportunity to provide genuine, and genuinely needed, help and support. In the pub, people I hardly knew would come over to ask about one thing or another, knowing I had 'had an education'. Later, when I earned some money from the media through discussing the study of the Milltown Boys, I spent it ostentatiously in the pub. In an anthropology module I had taken as an undergraduate, I had learned about the 'potlatch' of the Kwakiutl[84]: the more they gave away, the more their status was enhanced! I tried similar tactics. As early as 1978, I received £90.00 for doing a 50-minute interview with the *News of the World*, and £120.00 for an article in *New Society*. That bought a lot of drinks. As noted at the beginning of this book, BBC Radio 4 also paid me £120.00 for the radio programme they did about the Boys in May 1982; it was divided six ways – between Danny, Jerry, Pete, Ted, Marty and me. Pete recalled having "got some amount of money from you, when we did that thing for the BBC":

> I think that also a lot of people would have thought 'oh he's making a lot of money from writing these books and what did the Boys get out of it – well, it's pure exploitation', or it would have been … if you hadn't shared it round.

I was adamant I would not end up like Howard Parker, resented for seemingly having ripped them off. Instead, I was actually seen as rather smart, according to Denny's older brother, as he climbed into the car on the way to football one Sunday morning, having just seen my picture and read my interview in the *News of the World* (with the heading 'Stop making excuses for young crooks, they do it because it pays', even though – surprise, surprise – that was not exactly what I had said). The newspaper interview had been prompted by my article in *New Society* (itself largely constructed from a Sunday afternoon casual conversation with Marty), which had also been debated on the radio and which all the Boys already knew had paid me a lot of money, because I had made that very obvious as I bought everybody drinks in *The Wayfarer*.

> You're pretty clever really, aren't you, How. We tell you stuff in simple language. You put it into posh words and you get paid a fucking fortune for it. And then you talk to the paper about it, and get paid for that too, and then

---

84 The 'potlatch' was actually a gift-giving feast practised by the indigenous people of the west coast of north America (Canada and the USA), not just the Kwakiutl. It involved the giving away or destruction of wealth or valuable items in a display that re-affirmed an individual's leadership and power, and their connections to family, tribe and community.

they write it in simple words, so that we can read what we told you in the first place![85]

This was an amusing, yet very succinct analysis, if ever I heard one. I made a lot of effort to recycle the resources that accrued from the study of the Milltown Boys back in their direction, to be sure they never felt I had advanced my own career on their backs.

For the most part, I remained close to most of the Boys (though clearly not all – see below). Sometimes I had been the only one who visited them in custody. Parents said it was too far to go[86] or that they did not 'deserve' a visit! Some of the Boys may have joined the queue to buy me tickets to see Bob Dylan in 1978, but Dylan held no interest for them (although, as noted in Chapter 12, the extra-ordinary queue did stimulate Alex' curiosity, to the extent that he bought himself a ticket, and subsequent fandom of Dylan). David Bowie, on the other hand, did interest them. I bought six tickets for his Earls' Court concerts in 1978; I gave Marty, Pete and Gary a ticket each.

When I left Milltown for Birmingham in 1979, it was suggested that the Boys should pay me an annual visit on the first weekend every December. December 1st is Gary's birthday; hence the proposed date, as he was one of those with the idea. I never thought they would come, but they did, for four or five years, *en masse* – at least a dozen of them most times. Individuals also visited occasionally. Danny and his girlfriend looked after my house for a month when I went to America in 1980. A year after that, they came with me to see Dylan at the National Exhibition Centre near Birmingham. Danny continues to complain about that gig, because Dylan was deeply into his religious phase and played very few of his famous songs[87]. Less than two years later, in February 1983, soon after Danny was released from another custodial sentence, I was best man at their wedding.[88]

Weddings were one occasion when I really could reciprocate. As a photographer in a music venue (see Tristram 2014), I had some excellent cameras and lenses; I composed photo albums, as a wedding present, for a number of the Boys (namely Ted, Jerry, and Shaun). Years later, in 2000, when Denny married for the third time, I helped his eldest son prepare a best man's speech, at Denny's request. Denny told me it was going to be a small family gathering and I had asked why, therefore, was

---

85   There is a photograph of quite a number of the Boys, with me, in my house in Milltown, holding up a copy of the page in the *News of the World*. The Boys were immensely proud to be featured in the interview, if only by proxy.

86   Visiting Danny in Portland Borstal, Dorset, for a maximum of one hour, involved eight hours of sitting in a probation service minibus – four hours each way. And if there was an unexpected number of visitors, the length of the visit was sometimes unexpectedly reduced. Danny's parents never visited him there, though he served well over a year.

87   He only played mainly songs from his recent albums *Slow Train Coming* and *Saved*.

88   My best man's gift was an engraved silver Parker fountain pen with a thick italic nib. The pen is engraved as follows – Howard 19–2–83 Danny & Maria.

he inviting me? He said it was because, as an experienced public speaker, I could help his son prepare and practice his speech. That was the deal!

Did I go native? I always cite the war photographers who say that if you want to get a good picture, you've got to get close. I certainly got close. I certainly observed closely. I was given the opportunity to see the Boys close-up and I took it. Did I reveal everything I saw or learned? No. I was always very careful to distinguish between being in 'research mode' and being in 'friendship mode'. At the very beginning, it was neither. I was an accidental resident of Milltown, looking to be a volunteer in a youth club (a role I had played, elsewhere, before), where – in that role – I got to know the Boys. There were no plans for anything else. Two years later, however, I went into 'research mode', as I asked the Boys how they would feel about me 'hanging around' with them, going to court with them and visiting them in custody, in order to understand their lives and their perspectives on, and relationships with, the criminal justice system. As I got to know the Boys better, however, some (by no means all) of them started to confide in me about so much more. This propelled me into what might be called 'friendship mode': we were not 'friends' in any classic sense of the word (though, eventually, the likes of Danny, Spaceman and Gary became so). Pete, for example, came out as gay to me before anybody else. He had always questioned his sexuality, but was terrified of discussing it with anyone. He felt he could discuss it with me and he did so, coming out just a short while later to the rest of the Boys. Some of the Boys have continued to share other complex, deeper and more private thoughts with me. Why? As Paul said, having revealed a lot of deeply personal issues to me (which I have not mentioned in this book):

> Half the things I've been saying to you, well with most of the people I grew up with I wouldn't be saying it to them, because I wouldn't want to burden them. It's only because you are properly interested in ... well not just me, but all the Boys. I see the Boys, but how can I say to them what I say to you, some of the things I've told you ...? Well you're not going to talk about them ... With a lot of the Boys, it's just 'How are you?', 'Alright?', 'How's it going?'. They're good boys, don't get me wrong, but they don't want to listen to my problems, even when they know I've got them. Anyway, I always try to go around with a smile on my face. Like I've said to you, I can be up and I can be down, but they don't see me like that. And you know, most of the Boys from up the Rec, we've all had our ups and downs, but we don't like talking about it, not to other men, do you know what I mean? I talk to those two women I know, and I've been talking to you for an hour and a half, when I didn't know whether I'd be able to say anything. And it's made me feel better, talking to you. I've let a lot of things out to a fucking guy I haven't spoken to for 20 fucking years. I've let it all out ... you've always made me feel OK about telling you things.
>
> I was thinking about it the other day, after you called me to ask me to do this, and it wasn't just me but a lot of the Boys always said that they could talk to you. I've got your number now, 'cos I may want to talk to you again ...!

Despite Paul's warm words, there is a clue as to why the Boys are relaxed about talking to, and confiding in me: 'not to other men'. I am a useful repository for some of their deeper thoughts, experiences and behaviours, precisely because – paradoxically – I don't really count and don't really matter. It is precisely because I am *not* one of them that makes them more comfortable in sharing certain things with me.

At the same time, however, I do matter to them, too, and they matter to me: I do not go to birthday parties, weddings, funerals and other events to gather data for another book. I go because I am, partly, one of them. I enjoy their company. In fact, there are times when I feel more 'at home' with the Boys than I do with any other network of colleagues or friends. There is an authenticity – despite the lies – that I adore about them. I never laugh so much as when I am with them. They are phenomenally good company. So that is 'friendship mode'. When I want to 'do research', I tell them. I often ask them again about things I have heard or learned socially. It becomes clear very quickly whether or not they are willing to discuss them 'on the record'; there are times when they, very explicitly, say 'I want you to keep this to yourself' – probably a mixture of request and threat! Beyond what the Boys have told me on the record, primarily through the formal research interviews, I have often made use of general contextual information, harmless (and often amusing) stories and other anecdotes, but I have never revealed personal information or the *modus operandi* of individuals, criminal or otherwise. That approach, I believe, maintains my ethical integrity in a position of striking proximity to the Boys. And most of them trust me in that way.

In my interviews with them in 2020, I asked the Boys whether they could recall what they thought of me when I entered their lives and how that perception had changed over time. Gary had asserted that "well, you're part of us, you've been part of all of our lives". I was curious as to how others felt. My relationship with the Boys has certainly been unusual, to say the least. That was exactly how Pete described it – "unusual":

> Normally, this kind of work is done by people who come in from outside, into a community like ours, and they do their work, their research, for maybe six months, or it might be six years, and then they move on to the next thing, and move away … and you probably don't hear of them again. Whereas you're still around and you're still in contact … you've become a part of the story, really, haven't you? You were good to us in lots and lots and lots of very small ways. Like going to court. That was important to us, particularly for those, like me, who didn't have two parents or who didn't have a parent who'd attend with them. And just the space, you gave us what they'd call now a safe space, someone to talk to, who didn't judge us. And you were unique, in Milltown terms, certainly in my experience, because you came from outside, and because of your academic ability and your class difference, so you gave us different ways of thinking about the world. You gave us a vision of something outside, because you were the only one we knew from outside of the estate.

We were very lucky in that respect. Perhaps you didn't think about it like that, but that's certainly the way I would think about it. I think that's what a lot of the Boys got out of you. That's what a relationship is, isn't it; it cuts both ways.

Kelvin didn't even see the relationship as particularly unusual:

> I don't think we ever really saw you as an outsider. Obviously when you first came into our lives, at the youth club, you were obviously different to us, you know what I mean, but I always remember you as the easy-going type, happy to talk with us. We were comfortable with you. We could relate to you, that's the way I remember it. We could talk to you. We didn't feel threatened by you. You were different from the other youth workers up there. We were more comfortable with you.
>
> And we did think about things … I mean, you were a bit older than us, but no one ever thought it was strange. It wasn't that it was different times and that no one ever thought about those kinds of things, 'cos we did think about those things, because we knew, because they'd moved the priest at the church because he used to tickle you and touch you up, so we did know about it. We knew the difference between someone who was right and someone who was wrong, some of those we felt discomfort with and those we felt comfortable with, and you always fitted in the comfortable side. Otherwise we would never have let you get anywhere near us! Or put the other way, we would never have come anywhere near you. Some of us came to class you as a friend and we were blessed having you around. We might have been a bit naïve in those days, but we all had radars.

My relationship with the Boys had not always started like that. When Danny first set eyes on me, he took an instant dislike to me and often tells others that his first inclination was to "beat shit out of that posh-talking bastard". Having a rare weekend home leave from the approved school he was at, he had been restrained from doing so by some of the other Boys who already knew me (see below). Others remained suspicious of me for quite a long time, puzzled why somebody like me should be so inquisitive about their lives. After all, the culture on the estate was *not* to ask too many questions.

Paul captured the Boys' position on me rather well. Having been a "Rec-Boy through and through", he remembered *me* long before I would say that I knew *him*:

> Yeah, I can remember first of all the way you talked, and I thought 'Who's this dick here?' That's what I thought. But you know what, like you done for a lot of people, a lot of the Boys, you've fucking won them over. I mean, you do talk posh, but you must have had something in you, I wouldn't know what it fucking was, but obviously you cared about people, you cared about people like us, that's what I would say, and you fucking grew on everyone … slowly but surely!

In my research interview with Paul, we went on to talk about getting to know each other during his time, in the mid-1970s, on the Job Creation Programme, during which he commented, "I mean, even though we don't see each other, I'm glad you've been in my life".

Tony provided another measured view of how I connected to the Boys, as he recalled his early encounters with me:

> I don't have a vivid memory of the first time … it wasn't an epiphany about seeing this person we couldn't understand with a strange accent! What you've got to remember, Howard, is that you were young, but that we were that much younger. The age difference as you get older, well the years remain the same but the difference narrows. Then, you were that much older than us. You were good fun. You were still young and you were enthusiastic. I remember playing you at table tennis. Yes, I know you won! You were just a bit of an older lad. But we made a connection.
>
> You were an outsider, obviously, but we brought you in. And I think you got a fair rub of the green, hanging around with us! We allowed you in.
>
> No, I think you were – and still are, with the greatest respect – someone we know, not part of the inner sanctum, although we've never gone out to have an inner sanctum. I don't think there's ever been an intent not to let other people in. I suppose it's just *hard* really, for anyone to fully connect with us, because we've all known each other since we were five.
>
> You were half in, half out – yes, that's how I would see it. Because we did a lot of things that you didn't. And I'm glad you didn't. You'd have been in a lot of trouble if you had! So, you had the good sense to dip in and dip out, as and when. *We* let you join in some of the stuff we did and *you* decided what you wanted to join in. It's still the same, really. And most of us were quite happy with that.

Another quite fascinating and reflective perspective on my role and relationship with the Boys was expressed by Vic:

> Thinking about you, How, I never really looked at you as a stranger. All I remember is that you was another white guy but you was posh, you had a posh accent and you was a young guy learning about fucking reprobates in Milltown. Oh, I just thought he wants to learn about all of us fucking delinquents in Milltown, and I was just happy to go along with all that. You know, it wasn't about who you are or where you were fucking from; you were just a posh white guy who'd come to see us disadvantaged kids, that's all it was. In them days, you had the youth club and you had the youth club workers and I thought you were one of those.
>
> It was only really like later on, over the years, that I realised what you were doing in your life, that it was a bit more than that. You wanted to learn about us and how we lived our lives.

And uncannily echoing the thoughts of C. Wright Mills, Vic went on to say:

> and then I got to meet people who would say 'oh, fucking hell, how do you
> know Howard then …?' Like one time I was in [name of city centre pub]
> and there was two guys in there and they'd just finished their sociology
> course. They must have been in their twenties and we were in there having a
> drink and they were talking about crime and delinquency. So, I says to them
> that I know a fella who's into all that, and they said 'who?', and I mentioned
> your name and they said, 'fucking hell, we reads his work, how do *you* know
> him?' And I said, 'he's known me since I was a fucking kid. I said he used
> to come and watch us and learn … that's where he got all his knowledge,
> watching all us lot, 'cos we were fucking reprobates'! I said to them, 'that's
> what *you've* got to do, you've got to get out in the fucking field and learn
> about what goes on, not read about it just from a fucking book. You've got
> to get out there and mix. That's how you'll fucking learn'. And these guys –
> they were celebrating 'cos they'd just got their degrees – and these guys
> said they'd take note of that. And I said, 'well you should start by reading his
> fucking books', because I said he wrote books on all the Boys where I'm
> from, one when we were just grown up and one when we were middle-
> aged. They said, 'oh, we'll have to do that'. I never saw them ever again! Yeah,
> I said I knew Howard Williamson, and they said 'never' and I said, 'oh yes, he
> knows all the Boys'. I said, 'don't sit in an office, get out there in the field,
> with the real people. Then you'll get to know what really goes on in life.
> Otherwise you'll never learn'.

This was not, however, a view held by everybody in Milltown. Though reviews of
both *Five Years* and *The Milltown Boys Revisited* had been broadly complimentary,
and I had indeed talked about *The Milltown Boys Revisited* on Laurie Taylor's Radio
4 programme *Thinking Allowed* (in November 2004), there were one or two quite
unpleasant attacks.

As late as October 2009, there was a blog under the banner of 'Adventures in
Career Development' by somebody called Tristram Hooley. It lauded *The Milltown
Boys Revisited*, imagining it as a film:

> Reading the Milltown Boys Revisited I couldn't help but imagine it as a film.
> The characters/research subjects are so powerful that they leap off the page at
> you. So here is my 'treatment' of the opening moments of 'Miltown [*sic*] Boys
> The Movie'. Film 4 are welcome to use this for free!
>
> *The camera pans across a […] council estate and zooms in on a street emptying out
> of the local school. They are fighting and shouting as they head home or out to the rec.
> David Bowie's 'All the Young Dudes' plays in the background as the camera continues
> down the road passing by burnt out cars and broken windows before heading out into
> the woods behind the estate.*

We follow the camera through the woods as we see groups of young boys. The younger ones are playing in abandoned cars or stealing birds [sic] eggs, while the older ones sniff glue, smoke and drink.

Seasons change rapidly as we flash forward a few years. We see the same group of boys shoplifting, buying and selling drugs, heading off down the pub and painting the town red on Friday night. They argue, fight, pick up girls and live for kicks.

Flash forward twenty years as the strains of the Bowie track come to an end. Where are they now? Whatever happened to the Milltown Boys?

It is not often that an academic book conjures up a world and its inhabitants clearly enough for you to feel like you know them. The critical distance we usually employ in academic writing tends to reduce humanity to being bugs under our microscope. We observe trends, analyse facts and figure [*sic*] and maybe even make policy recommendations. However it is a rare book that hums with the life and humanity that normally characterise a good novel. *The Milltown Boys Revisited* is one of those books and I'd argue that almost everyone would get something out of reading it. However, for those interested in career, learning and the role of guidance the book is even more essential.

(Hooley 2009)

Hooley goes on to describe the book in more detail and to draw some implications for career guidance. He concludes with the remark that 'All in all this is a fantastic book. It doesn't provide us with a lot of answers, but it certainly asks a lot of interesting question [*sic*]'.

I had not seen the blog at the time but when I was preparing for *this* book, I discovered it by chance. Having read the plaudits, I perused the comments that followed. None was posted for a year! The first, that appeared in December 2010, suggests that I am 'a bit stereotypical' and that my 'discourse appears to be a bit judgemental'. The second expresses interest in that reaction, suggesting instead that I had 'a really strong empathy with the "boys"'. This led to the first person say that she would elaborate on her arguments 'as soon as I finish the book!'.

The fourth comment, however, posted anonymously one and a half years after the first three, in March 2012, is brutal towards me:

Howard Williamson was a snake in the grass, I've met lot of the "boys" talked about in the book and even Williamson himself all he did was use the "boys" for a book ... sounds totally ridiculous how Williamson had planned to write the book all along but he did. Williamson likes to command his image as somewhat of a working-class hero. I find it quite frankly hilarious when people say he spent years "researching" the "boys" he was sniffing glue with them. i saw one of the "boys" talked in the book recently he expressed his annoyance on how Williamson had used them. Pretending to be their friends with a plan to write a book all along. [He] had also told me how Howard Williamson had always told him how he wanted to be in TV some day. I mean seriously a person researching "Juvenile Delinquents" who shared dreams of Television presenting with one of the "boys" Trust me guys what may seem an insightful book about issues of youth crime is just little snippets of a typical council estate. I feel the people who think this book is controversial and shocking really haven't lived at all …

When I first read this, perhaps understandably, I felt quite deeply hurt, though not so much because of the attack on me, however vindictive it seemed to be, but because it was so dreadfully *wrong*. I had never intended to write a book about the Boys. Things had unfolded in an almost accidental and incremental way as I seized on circumstances and opportunities. I had moved to Milltown quite by chance in 1973. I had volunteered as a youth worker on a run-down 'adventure playground', known locally as 'the club'. As I have outlined already, that was primarily where I developed my connections and relationships with the Boys. It was only two years later that I consulted with them about exploring their experiences of the criminal justice system, to which they agreed. This specific focus became the theme for my postgraduate studies but, through my participant observation with the Boys, I obviously learned a great deal more than that. As a result, when I left Milltown in 1979, I quietly wrote a memoir of my time on the estate, feeling that I had had a privileged insight into the lives of the Boys and I did not want to forget. It was a private and personal recollection. Only some while later did an academic colleague[89] ask me if I had ever written about my time in Milltown, and I sent her a copy of the memoir. She thought it was good and suggested I should try to get it published. This was what became *Five Years*. Of course, I did plan to write a second book, though the idea to do so only came to me towards the end of the 1990s. It was written with the full consent of those of the Boys who are included in it. All of this is carefully explained in *The Milltown Boys Revisited* (pp.17–23). I certainly never told anyone of aspirations to work in TV, because I never had any! And I have never sniffed glue (though I did sometimes come across the Boys in the woods, some of whom were high on glue, and indeed I have photographs of them doing so).

On the same day as the accusatory comment was posted, there was a comment from the moderator, who had already removed some content from the tirade against me (material that 'compromised the anonymity of one of the "boys"'), expressing uncertainty about how to respond to the anonymous accusatory remarks. The moderator went on, 'I don't want to get involved in a flame war here and I'm happy to host a range of opinions on this blog. Is this the right approach?' A moderator for a different blog replied less than an hour later that, if the comment had been made on her blog, 'it would not have got through moderation unless it had come from a named individual with whom I could have had a discussion about the reason(s) for the comment'. She also questioned whether there had ever been any claim that the

---

89 This was Dame Professor Teresa Rees CBE, who became a lifelong friend and who, over many years in the 1980s, supported my rather *ad hoc* university employment through a sequence of short-term research contracts.

book was 'controversial and shocking'. The moderator of the blog responded that they were trying to keep an unmoderated blog, to only 'take stuff down when it is clearly spam or offensive' and conceding that the comment in question is 'sort of in the borderland between legitimate comment and offensiveness. That's why I'm not sure what to do'.

As noted, I was rather upset by the arguably offensive comment and, as I read through the rest of them, including a short supportive comment in May 2014 by 'Gary Milltown' ("Was both sad and exciting but fair … Gary MIlltownboys"), I reached the last one, posted astonishingly as late as July 2015, over three years after the contentious comment:

> The former anon description of Howard Williamson as a "Snake in the grass" is quite risible and largely formed from hearsay, considering he trusted and invited many self-confessed thieves and hooligans (myself included) into his life and into his home without anything being touched or stolen.
>
> I was one of those "hooligans" and the only reptilian qualities I ever detected from Howard was a lovely faux crocodile skin belt he used to wear. Everybody is entitled to their opinions though and I can say that I knew Howard from the time he first stepped into Milltown up until two days ago when I last saw him (41 years?) and he never did me no wrong.
>
> The book, in my opinion was spot on and although there are a few things he says about me which I don't quite agree with, it is nevertheless his truth, and just as valid as if I were to write "my truth" about Howard and his illustrious cohorts.
>
> I thoroughly recommend the book to any students of sociological subjects, or an interest in the social structures within our society. A glimpse into how society treats it's [sic] working class youth, and the struggles and frustrations inherent with those caught within "The exclusion zone".
>
> Good read – give it a go.

The comment was signed off by 'Spaceman, Milltown'! If anyone understands my character, and my motives and motivations for writing about the Boys, he does.

Even the Boys (and their siblings) were not always so effervescent as Vic was about me to the two sociology graduates in the pub. Right from the start, there were moments that caused considerable discomfort, if not outright fear. At Ted's first wedding (where I was the photographer), surrounded by his mainly older brothers and sisters, one older brother with a formidable reputation suddenly commented, referring to *Five Years*, that "it wasn't so nice what you wrote about our kid". The remark killed the atmosphere and there was a tense silence in the air. I looked anxiously for the exit door. Ted's family did not mess about or hang on ceremony. Then Ted's matriarchal older sister, Rhian (see Chapter 7), broke the ice and said "It wasn't nice, but it was all true". The brothers calmed down but it was not until Ted's younger sister's funeral, which Ted had explicitly asked me to attend, that the extended family really came to acknowledge that, *despite* my sometimes rather damning portrayal of Ted, there was a longstanding positive relationship between us.

Many years later, Tony cornered me at another gathering, long after the publication of *The Milltown Boys Revisited*. He told me he was quite deeply unhappy with my portrayal of his impoverished childhood and his single mother. He made the point that he had been, with his next youngest sibling, the *beneficiary* of single parenthood, whereas his older brothers and sisters had grown up in a household with a violent, abusive father and suffered accordingly in a variety of ways. Tony was not angry with me – indeed, during the conversation, he bought me another drink – but felt that I had not struck the right chord on that part of his portrait, though he was otherwise rather pleased with the way I had depicted him elsewhere in the book.

Even in the early years, I met many of the Boys' parents and older relatives, sometimes just by chance in the shops or on the bus, but sometimes in their houses. Pete's mother, with a cigarette permanently between her lips and ash dropping on to the floor, invited me in for a cup of tea. Jerry's father, as I have noted already, often asked me to raise a glass of whisky with him at Christmas time. Danny's uncle Greg – a removal man – used his van to transport my possessions to Birmingham when I moved from Milltown in April 1979. Marty's grandmother was always welcoming to me, often inviting me in for a cup of tea or even something to eat; many years later, her eyesight and hearing failing, I went to see her but she didn't answer the door when I rang the bell. I saw her through the window and tapped on it; without hesitation, she told me to come round the back. Only after she had made me a cup of tea, when she called me 'Daniel', did I realise that she had thought I was Marty's brother, though even when I confirmed who I really was, she was still quite happy to make me welcome. But it had not always started like that, as Mark noted:

> Well you were the bloke up the rec, helping to run the youth club. That's what I remember first about you. But I think, more than anything, our parents were wary of you; you know, they were probably thinking what's this bloke doing hanging around with kids, you know what I mean. But I remember you walking in the rec, into the club, and like all of us, we were thinking who's this fucking dude, what does he want?
>
> But when you look back, you helped us to have a place to go. It was a place where you wasn't criticised, where you didn't have a go at us, do you get my meaning? You didn't look at us like we were fucking animals, you know, thugs and delinquents, you sort of treated us like normal people, you know, and that's the best way I can describe it. And that way you got our respect.
>
> And you used to come to court and talk to my mum. I think she was, like the others, a bit wary at first, you know, 'who's this bloke?', or whatever, but as time went on, my mum used to say 'he's a nice man, that Howard, isn't he?' and I think she'd tell a lot of the other parents the same.

The very first 60th birthday party held by one of the Boys (though not one included explicitly in my previous books) took place in 2019. Quite a few of the Boys met up in a pub beforehand. I joined them there. They were, as usual, very welcoming. But during the laughs and witty repartee, Gary's older sister Jacqui asked me how I had got to know the Boys. She is about three years older than Gary and, as a teenager, she had been a hard, skinhead girl, reminiscent of Vicky McClure's character (Lol) and image in Shane Meadows' *This is England*, a realist portrayal of rough working-class racist Britain. She had become a successful businesswoman, setting up her own social care company. In the pub, she revealed that she had always been "a bit suspicious" of me. I had found this very disconcerting. After all, I knew Gary very well, had taken him to see David Bowie in 1978, had known his parents and had known *her* all those years ago. Jacqui said she knew exactly who I was but had never been able to fathom out what I had wanted. What exactly had I been doing when I had been hanging around with her younger brother? Where had I come from? How had I ended up in Milltown? We spent much of the evening continuing the conversation at the party, interspersed with many of the other Boys coming over to say it was good that I had come. At the end of the night, Jacqui apologised for having had such doubts and wondered whether a farewell hug might still be in order. I thanked her for the chat, saying that I really appreciated that *finally* we had cleared the air – after nearly 50 years! We had the hug.

The Boys do recognise my place in their lives, as I do theirs in mine. As I scrolled through the news feed on Facebook in 2017, I came across the cover image of *The Milltown Boys Revisited*. Mack had posted it with the caption "Just read this book about me and the boys great read". It triggered quite an exchange between different people from Milltown. One of the 'avenue Boys' asked if he could get a copy; Mack said he had got his "£10 e bay" and added "It's a book about the rec boys". Like a flash, another of the avenue boys chipped in "So it's only one page then" and a woman whose name I did not recognise wrote "Not about the rec girls then xx", adding, when Mack replied "No lol", "Aghhh they don't know what they missed pmsl"[90]. Somebody else noted that they had read the first book and "would like to read the follow up book"; Mack offered to lend it and said they would sort it out in the week. Another 'avenue Boy' asked Mack "wots Millbank [*sic*] got to do with us lads up the Rec", to which Mack replied that "Howard had to change the names". After a considerable number of comments like this, I joined in, explaining why I had not including the stories of the girls nor accounts from the 'avenue Boys'. And I corrected 'Millbank', explaining that I had called the area 'Milltown', given the estate's connections to the local paper mill.

Facebook has been the repository of many interesting, and sometimes revealing, words and pictures. One of Ted's daughters posted a picture of Ted and me on one of my visits, with the caption "nice visit from the prof", to which another of the Boys wrote "A blast from the past nice", while somebody else noticed I had a star above my head (it was Christmas time) which attracted the comment "he's always

90 In case the text speak is lost on the reader: 'pissed my-self laughing'.

been a star", and the younger of Ted's two older sisters, who had apparently visited later the same day, wrote "Sorry to have missed you Howard it would have been lovely to have seen you x".

So, although there have to be some caveats, I generally feel vindicated with the approach I have taken over the years in relation to the Boys. I have endeavoured to balance a 'research' and 'friendship' relationship with them and, for the most part, it seems to have worked.

It wasn't even easy to finalise a research interview with Danny, with whom perhaps I have had the closest relationship over the years. He had had no objection to being interviewed and I knew he would have plenty to say. But recurrent WhatsApp video conversations, though they covered some of the ground, failed to nail down a suitable date, largely because Danny was nearly always taking care of his grandson, even during the Covid-19 lockdown. Almost every day he was out with Alfie, either over the woods or by the river, playing games, climbing trees and fishing. Even when we did eventually agree on a date, I called him and got no answer. Not long afterwards I got a text:

> Okay mate can we arrange for another day got plenty on at the moment …
> will be in touch soon … Milltown worrior

I cryptically wrote back that I thought he meant 'warrior'; I was the worrier! Less, surprisingly, the following day, my planned research interview with Paul was postponed. He, too, sent me a text: "Can I leave today Howard. My heads in the shed, phone you in a couple of days". Just a few days later, he did; worried that if I called him, he might not even answer his phone (which was his habit on his 'down' days), he had a few drinks and sent me another text: "Phone me when ready. Not too late. lol". I did not pass up the opportunity and had started my research interview with Paul less than ten minutes later. Danny called me soon after that, and my final, 12th, research interview was concluded. Both of them honoured their word.

It is telling that Danny was my final research respondent. With perhaps the exception of Spaceman over the past 20 years, he is the one with whom I have maintained closest contact. That was certainly the case over the previous 25 years. I had been best man at his wedding in 1983, an event that had had to be postponed twice because he had been in custody. He eventually got married ten days after being released from an 18-month prison sentence.

I used the research interview not only to follow the topic guide I had used in my interviews with all the other Boys but also to probe and question, in finer detail, some of the nuances of their accounts. In particular, I was interested in how we had somehow struck up a lifelong relationship, given his place on the criminogenic extreme amongst the Boys and mine in the realms of professional respectability:

> Straight away, I saw you as 'authority'. I came up the club with Richard and
> I was sat on the bench in the club. I was on home leave from approved school
> and I saw you, and you were asking questions. And my immediate thoughts

were that the sort of questions you were asking reminded me of the fucking probation or the police, you know what I mean. So, I said to somebody, I can't remember who it was, 'who's that over there?' And they said, 'oh, that's Howard, he's a sociologist, and I didn't know what that was'. And I remember thinking, if he comes over here and starts asking me fucking questions he's going to get my fucking fist in his face. And then when it was nearly time to go, you came over and spoke to me, and I thought he's quite pleasant, really … you were easy going. The first time I came over your flat, I was mesmerised by all your records, and all your tapes and photos and books and everything. And I thought this man's alright, this man is what it's all about, really … and that was it, really. You had a lot of respect from the Boys. Yeah, we had a lot of respect for you.

And then, later, I wanted you to be my best man because you were the sensiblist person I knew. You made things happen, I knew you were the one I could trust. By that time, we got on so well. I'd been to your house in Birmingham. Yeah, we [he and Maria] talked about it and we both thought you'd be the best person for us when we got married, if you were willing to do it. I liked you. I thought a lot of you, that's how it was. And I bought you that fountain pen – yes, I *bought* it – as a thank you. And I know my parents were so pleased that we'd got to know each other.

On the evening before Danny's wedding, I slept on the floor in the box-room of his parents' council house. Just under 40 years later, as the Covid-19 lockdown eased, I went for a long walk in the woods with Danny and his grandson. If that does not convey some notion of the 'distant intimacy' that characterises this study, I am not quite sure what would.

15

SOME FINAL THOUGHTS

The Milltown Boys grew up at a certain time, and in a certain place. They came from a distinctive social class and culture and were from a particular post-war generation. Many were born into what later came to be depicted as the 'underclass', a deeply contested and controversial concept. As I argued in a discussion of 'status zer0' youth (Williamson 1997), which most of the Boys passed through at one point or another in their transitions to adulthood, there are questions as to whether there really is a category that reflects stable members of what might be called an underclass, rather than one that can describe unstable members of the working-class. The Boys' parents certainly fell into the latter group: most worked, at least for most of the time, but their work was often, in fact usually, casual, precarious and unpredictable. They were not the beneficiaries of the more regulated and remunerated labour markets that prevailed for many working-class people in the post-war era, within the public sector and through the strength of the trade union movement. They were generally poorly paid, and many of the Boys testified to growing up poor (see Davin 1996).

The Boys themselves became extremely vulnerable to the first major post-War recession, officially leaving school in the mid-1970s. Those were the days of the first government youth training programmes (the Job Creation Programme and the Youth Opportunities Programme), to ease the transition from school to work. Those who struggled to get a foothold in the labour market would, today, be viewed as afflicted with 'scarring effects' (see Bell and Blanchflower 2011), though this was not known at the time: the disproportionately negative lifetime effects of early unemployment. Indeed, one of the 'killer facts' produced for a British government review of young people's lives, drawn from the 1970 Birth Cohort Study (i.e. children born a decade after the Boys), was that those who were 'status zer0' or latterly described as not in education, employment or training ('NEET') in 1986 (at age 16) were some 8.5 times more likely to be unemployed in 1996 (at the age of 26) (see Social Exclusion Unit 2000).

On the other hand, there was, at least in theory, greater opportunity open to the Boys. They did not, as Marty had put it, have to be 'stifled' by their own past. There was the possibility of progress, choice and mobility, to some extent at least. Tony moved away. Pete came out as gay and went to London. Kelvin became a photographer. Shaun got an apprenticeship. Gordon embraced entrepreneurship. The Boys were not pre-destined to become casual labourers and to break the law.

But many, indeed most, did end up in unskilled occupations and/or on the wrong side of the law. Was this the outcome of their class position or their cultural inheritance? Was it because of some criminogenic apprenticeship or generational continuity? Why did only a few of the Boys who left Milltown never come back? Why did many never leave? There are never clear answers but any answer is likely to need to accommodate different elements of many of these factors and the way in which they exerted influences in different directions. The 'pushes' and 'pulls' at play should not, indeed cannot, be underestimated. Tony was pulled away by a more attractive job offer, but would he have gone had his wife not been pushing in the same direction? Vic was pulled towards professional rugby league in the north of England, but there was no one to push him to stay there, and he came home. Professional and occupational 'pulls' and 'pushes' in the working environment (whichever side of the law) have to be weighed with and against those exerted more personally and privately in the domestic arena. And the relative influence of different pressures also ebbs and flows over time, as some arenas of life become more stable and settled, while others become more volatile and uncertain. Either way, sometimes these are intrinsically established, whereas at other times they are externally imposed. The imposition of a home detention curfew on Danny compelled him to do some legitimate work with his brother; Mack's wife threatened to throw him out if he continued using whizz (speed); Gary left home because of deteriorating relationships there; and the 'affray' case for a number of the Boys was a 'wake-up call' to put some legitimate order into their lives.

The one really lucky break afforded to a significant minority of the Boys, one which, for most of those to whom it was made available, gave them some stability and order, was the right-to-buy scheme introduced by Margaret Thatcher in the 1980s. Designed to promote a 'property-owning democracy', it enabled quite a few of the Boys to get on to the private housing ladder so that, paradoxically, in 2020, when most young people – including many from far more privileged backgrounds – are struggling with their housing costs, many of the Boys (though by no means all) are sitting rather comfortably on considerable housing assets. Not one of them had grown up in private housing.

With regard to transitions to the labour market, the story of the Boys suggests the need for a great deal of caution in conducting short-term research on cohorts as they leave school. Concluding that things become 'settled' by the late teens or early 20s produces false and misleading comfort and confidence, in view of episodes later in life. Scarring may generate ongoing and long-term precarity; security is never guaranteed. Job losses, relationship breakdown, physical and mental health problems can quickly catapult individuals into much more vulnerable positions, in relation to offending, housing, health and relationships. Trevor, for example, having once determined that he would never offend again, reverted to crime for a short while, when he lost his job: after all, he knew the right people and he knew what to do. For many more people today, circumstances are imbued with greater risk; the Milltown Boys were arguably at the vanguard of those vulnerabilities, however much they sought to stabilise their situation, one way or another. In that sense, their stories provide something of a litmus test for things to come, for marginalised young people in precarious situations in any social context.

Many of the Boys did stabilise their situation far more than might have been anticipated – one way or another. That they found a way through is, in some respects, quite remarkable. That around a third did so on the right side of the tracks, even rather successfully, is particularly impressive. Given the collapse of industry and the loss of any possibility of following in the footsteps of their fathers (the 'lads of dads' syndrome – see Lee and Wrench 1983), or even their older brothers, it really is quite surprising that rather more of the Boys did not fall by the wayside, succumbing to profound social exclusion, even if some of them did – later, if not sooner.

The peer group certainly held things together, even in times of considerably adversity, for many of the Boys. As we have seen, they have remained wedded to each other (not quite literally!), almost irrespective of the paths taken throughout their lives. This has enabled them to sustain a level of resilience that can easily take people by surprise. Given precarious employment, often fragile domestic relationships (with partners and with children), physical and mental health issues, and (for some) the ever-present threat of criminal justice interventions, it is surprising just how robust and resilient the Boys have generally continued to be.

To some extent at least, this has also been forged on the anvil of a very narrow conception of time and a limited perspective on space. The Boys are reluctant to look too far back and resistant to looking too far forward. The past is sometimes hard to acknowledge and memories are not always rosy (for either the Boys or those whom they have affected, in many different ways); the future is unknown and perhaps too risky to imagine, especially for those still embroiled in criminal activity or those with health conditions. The Boys are intrinsically fatalistic – as noted above (footnote 80) and as they themselves would say, 'what's done, is done', and 'qué sera, sera'.

The vast majority of the Boys have also stayed on, or very close to their 'patch', even if this conceals considerable geographical mobility at earlier points in their lives. But Milltown is where they feel 'at home'. It is their home. It is where they draw strength, through familiarity and connection. They know the place and people know them. We have learned, in this text, that many of the Boys have, however, withdrawn more into their homes, even those with a 'name' on the street; a number commented that there was too much of a desire amongst the younger generation to take them on. This is an interesting observation, because many of the benefits accruing from their identity *in Milltown* may only now be starting to dissipate and unravel. In other words, what has sustained them so far may soon evaporate. Only Ted has built a similar support structure in another place. Of the other Boys who have left, Pete and Shaun have retreated into self-isolation (both, in part, on account of a combination of relationships issues and mental health problems). Richard is in a similar predicament, for the same reasons, though he lives on an adjacent estate and does return to Milltown quite regularly. Derek was never completely part of Milltown and, now living on the other side of the city, sees the Boys less and less. In contrast, Matt, Spaceman, Alex and Jamie, who also don't live far away, retain strong connections with the area, through the Boys. Tony and Gordon have established more middle-class lifestyles, but they too have sustained their social connections with the Boys, appearing in Milltown for social events, from time to time.

Life for most of the Boys moves forward on that basis – a narrow window of time and firmly anchored in or near to Milltown – and it has taken significant events or experiences to produce any radical shift in direction, some of which proved to be temporary (through choice or circumstance), while some turned out to be more permanent. Jamie's white-collar job, to 'tide him over Christmas' in 1996 is the seminal case in point; he is still there! But there are many other, quite invisible, examples. Trevor's football injury – which left him, after a series of operations, with one leg shorter than the other, until he discovered that he could get an 'elevator shoe' like 'Rocky'[91] – meant he could no longer be a milkman[92] and he had to rethink his occupational pathway. It was only Shaun's marriage breaking up that propelled him into becoming the student of electrical engineering and obtaining the university degree he had always dreamed of; though after getting it, he resumed work as an electrician. More recently, Vic went back to work, painting ships, to escape a fractured relationship.

These were all examples of what Giddens (1991) has called 'fateful moments', which were sometimes built into the fabric of the life-course (precarious work, atrophying relationships, physical injuries) and sometimes enshrined the shock of the unexpected. The latter were what the Boys themselves sometimes referred to as 'wake-up time', something that aroused them from the stupor of their everyday routines and propelled them towards something different. Kelvin may not have viewed some serious fighting in town as a criminal act until he found himself in Crown Court staring – if found guilty – a prison sentence in the face. That concentrated his mind about fighting in the future. Spaceman might never have contemplated going to Art College (and moving on to getting a degree) had his probation officer not complimented him on his drawings and suggested he could make something of himself.

---

91 Sylvester Stallone increases his height by some inches through wearing Chamaripa 'elevator shoes'.

92 Trevor had a milk round franchise with Unigate, in Milltown, and – as a fast runner – was able to catch and 'sort out' kids who tried to steal from his milk float. After his dreadful ankle injury, incurred playing football, he could no longer catch them, resulting in the loss of many pints of milk, no income and dramatic occupational reorientation – to sitting down, driving HGV vehicles, for the next ten years. He has remained self-employed and now fits uPVC windows.

Without fateful moments and wake-up time, were the Boys ploughing their own furrow or stuck in a rut? After knowing them for almost 50 years, it is still difficult to say.

Feral or free?

Throughout much of their lives, most of the Boys have continued to live with a strong sense of autonomy and libertarianism. So long as no one gets in their way, they let others 'do their thing'. But they insist on being able to do theirs and, when people get in the way, they have tried to push them to one side. When they have been unable to do that, they have taken the consequences, let things take their course, and continued with their own preferred lifestyles as soon as they have been able to. This applies as much to those who have been relatively successful on the right side of the tracks (like Tony, Gordon or Jamie) as to those who have not fared so well on the wrong side of the tracks (like Nathan, Eddie, Mack and Paul). And for those in the middle – one side or the other – or for those swinging from one side *to* the other (like Matt or Vic), they have made the best of things when the chances have arisen, and fatalistically accepted things that have worked against them.

Rarely have the Boys complained deeply about the inequalities or injustices that, arguably, have shaped and framed their lives in ways that have dealt them a poor hand. Only when personal or institutional decisions have affected contact with their children have they articulated a sense of grievance, as we have seen in the more recent circumstances of Vic and Matt, and as was experienced much earlier in life by Paul and Denny.

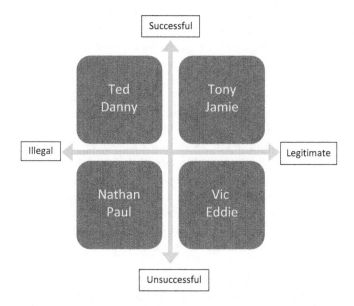

FIGURE 15.1 Examples of the Boys' *economic* life-course and lifestyle pathways

When I first wrote about the Milltown Boys, I described their teenage lives as being 'out of sight, out of mind' (though, paradoxically, I noted that it was also important for the Boys to be *seen*): nobody had any real idea about what they were doing, nor did anybody apparently seem to care. Most really were out on the street, from dawn to dusk, often 'mitching' (skiving) school and just hanging around, in town, on the estate or in the woods. Matt made a telling remark:

> I feel sorry for the kids today. I feel sorry for anyone who's in their 40s, 30s, 20s and that. We were lucky. We were the last ones who lived on the street. We had our freedom. Today everybody's been brainwashed, told what they can do, and what they can't do. We just did whatever we wanted to … We were mad, we were crazy, but we were free … We were wild and free.

There was certainly a feral streak in many of the Boys that was enabled, perhaps even caused, by that freedom. In their youth, there was no doubt that they were 'wild boys', getting into all kinds of mischief, violence and trouble – living for today – without any thought of penalties or consequences. Ted freely admitted that, whether it was in the children's homes or in the workplace, he "couldn't take the discipline", and routinely fought back. Spaceman would probably say that it was their 'punk' mentality: *No Future*, as the Sex Pistols put it and as Cashmore (1984) analysed it.

Whether or not that was the primary catalyst for their 'devil may care' attitude and approach to life, the Boys certainly exercised 'agency' (active self-determination) far more than their structural position might have suggested they would or could (see Williamson 2021). Arguably, they might often have been wiser to engage in more compromise and concession – with partners, in the workplace and on the street. Instead, they were rarely prepared to put up with 'shit', as they defined it, and either walked (not ran) away or fought back, classic flight or fight responses designed to preserve their autonomy and sense of dignity. The consequences when they fought back were often dire for them – imprisonment, restraining orders, dismissal from work, loss of contact with children, the collapse of relationships, sometimes homelessness, loss of income, and more. But, and here is a paradox once again, if it did not destroy them (as it did Marty and Eddie and, later, Richard and Nathan, through mental ill-health, addiction or premature physical decline), they continued to hold their heads high. They were determined to do so. Even some of those who have fallen on really hard times, including Nutter, have preserved their sense of autonomy by retreating into the woods, where they live for much of the year in tents, holding what the Boys told me was a 'never ending party' fuelled by alcohol and drugs. As one of them described it, "They're all down there on the weekend and some are there nearly all the time. It's like a palace and a pub rolled into one, under canvas".

The Boys had little faith that either religion or politics would come to their rescue. They largely believed that they were on their own in this world; all the more reason, they said, for banding together and retaining strength in numbers. Some, like Jamie, did assert explicitly that they were "Labour through and through", had always voted and could never vote for 'them' (Conservatives) on the grounds that that would be betraying their working-class roots. Yet significant numbers of them had voted for the UK to leave the European Union in the Referendum of 2016, albeit for very different reasons, and many had voted for the Conservatives and Boris Johnson in the General Election of 2019, largely in order to 'get Brexit done'. Most of the Boys, however, vehemently rejected politics and religion, convinced that these were games to be played by others, and they were not going to be pawns in those games, though some had been in their younger days – foot-soldiers for the Socialist Workers Party and the National Front, abused by Catholic priests. They knew the social order did not operate in their favour, that those in power looked after themselves; there was little they could do about it, except to try, whichever way they could, to look after *themselves*.

When discussing his 'time' in the Merchant Navy, in prison and at university, Spaceman – who, in many respects, was the archetypical existential libertarian amongst the Boys – reflected philosophically that they had all "stamped their institutional experience on me":

> They're all the same really. You become a number and you have to do your time. They're all forms of control. You're part of their captive audience. They keep records on you and you have to do what you're told, until they set you free. It don't matter whether you're a sailor, a prisoner or a student – you're trapped and you're not you …

Spaceman put up with it, in the first place (the Merchant Navy) because he didn't know any better, in the second (prison) because he had no choice, and in the third (university) "because art college is a place for pop stars – they all went to art college – and I wanted a bit of that magic", but he resented and resisted his loss of freedom, fighting back through drinking, breaking the rules and producing his own chosen brand of art: "I always wanted to stamp my view on the world". Matt put it more succinctly: "I've done so much wild things all through my life that I don't really know what normal life is".

The individualisation thesis much loved by sociologists did not resonate with the Boys. Their personal agency was possible only through their collective identity. No one else was likely to stand up for them, but they could – and would always – stand up for each other.

New times, old ways?

In *The Milltown Boys Revisited*, quite a number of the Boys were concerned, that their children (cf. their sons) might grow up too 'soft', lacking the hard and street-wise edge that they themselves had acquired through growing up on the street. Ideally, they wanted their kids to develop characteristics that somehow combined the cultural strengths of the Boys' deprived childhoods with the wider social opportunities with which they were now presented. They were usually proud when their children (usually unexpectedly) secured educational and sporting achievements, and reasonably accepting when those individuals (notably the daughters of Danny and Tommy) did not sustain them. They did not express too much disappointment when their children seemed to be following in their footsteps. After all, at the time, few felt they were in any position to do anything about it.

Twenty years further on, as the occupational paths of the Milltown Boys have polarised yet further, one can now discern a different kind of combination of prospects for their now adult children, one that embraces modern times through making use of old methods of contacts and possibility. Once again, this applies to life-course pathways on both sides of the tracks. Gary's daughter works for his sister's social care company. Both of Tony's daughters work for him. Jamie's son got into his professional career through a fellow skittles player. In the more shadowy world of crime and drugs, Vic's son from his second relationship is an 'entrepreneur' who works closely with Ted's oldest son, from his first relationship. Generationally, therefore, they are all still looking out for one another, by means of their own sustaining 'social capital' – the networks that have kept them going through good times and bad (see Putnam 2000).

Trajectories or navigations?

In 1997, Karen Evans and Andy Furlong published an important article on 'metaphors of youth transitions' (Evans and Furlong 1997). They debated whether youth transitions were best considered as niches, pathways, trajectories or navigations. In reality, they are something of all of these, which is powerfully emphasised by the life stories of the Boys. Jamie was 'slotted in', finding an unexpected niche in a workplace he never thought he would experience. Gary followed a pathway into a line of work and way of thinking that was shaped, though not determined, by his father. Indeed, Gary would be the first to concede that he might have gone in other directions. Paul was launched into a lifetime of substance dependency and 'social exclusion'; his trajectory was heavily framed by the weight of a trio of adverse teenage experiences – a lack of educational participation, incessant substance misuse and the acquisition of a protracted criminal record. He might say that it has been "all my fault", but others might disagree. Trevor has navigated his way through various challenging moments during his life and, each time, emerged for the better: a 'wake up' moment while being held in a police cell, a reconsideration of his occupational future after the traumatic football injury that left him with one leg shorter than the other, and the tactical exchange of a council house on which he subsequently exercised his right-to-buy.

There is also always a significant academic debate about the balance of 'agency' and 'structure' in influencing the life course of individuals. To what extent do they lack 'life management' and are they 'knocked around by uncontrollable forces' (see Helve and Bynner 1996) rather than applying what Swartz and Cooper (2014) have referred to as 'navigational capacities' (see also Swartz 2021)? How much did the

Boys succumb to the 'risk society' (Beck 1992) or develop what Evans (1998) has called 'constrained agency'?

We have to take great care in imputing either active self-determination or passive acquiescence to any of the Boys. Within the niches, pathways, trajectories and navigations referred to above, there were moments *across* the life course and within different parts of their lives *at the same time* when different levels of autonomy and passivity came to bear. When Spaceman moved house, he made sure that it was to an apartment with plenty of roof space for his art work. Vic, whose public persona is of a strong, 'hard', assertive individual, literally broke down in the face of what he viewed as impenetrable bureaucracy and discrimination against absent fathers. Few of the Boys have been eternally or incessantly knocked around from pillar to post, nor have many of the Boys clearly and confidently driven their lives forward completely through their own volition.

It might be preferable to consider life course decisions in terms of whether the Boys have been proactive or reactive, and – in relation to each decision – how much room for manoeuvre, of which they were aware, was available to them. Going to prison might suggest little scope for 'agency' of any kind, yet the collective knowledge (even wisdom) about custody amongst the Boys meant that most were well prepared for the experience and already had contacts and networks on the inside when they got there. That helped considerably in the balance of power within the prison system. Similar points can be made in relation to the social security system, with which many of the Boys have been dealing throughout their lives. They have a wealth of experience as to how to maximise receipt of benefits, while minimising the burden of expectations and controls imposed on them.

Nonetheless, it is invariably some combination of external circumstance and internal judgment that moved the Boys in particular directions. Gary had two critical moments – being banned from *The Wayfarer* that propelled him towards the 'catholic' Boys, and then staring prison in the face when on trial for affray and actively deciding that 'enough was enough' and that it was time to change course and buckle down. Mark, too, was excluded from *The Wayfarer* because, at the age of 16, he looked too young (he *was* too young, but most of his mates of the same age were still allowed in, and got served). Instead, he was enrolled by his father in the social club. Having hated school ("all I ever wanted to do was earn some money") he'd got a job as a porter in a city centre hotel, while the rest of the Boys were either unemployed or working in the local fruit market. Mark was earning "about £7.00 a week more than most of them and much more than they were getting on the dole". He says this gave him choices the other Boys did not have, without stealing! He had the money for going to watch the football and to buy a drink (in the social club). Football, however, through the violence so deeply associated with it at the time, still got him into trouble (see *The Milltown Revisited*, p.57) and he needed a sharper 'wake-up call':

> I hated the fucking coppers who nicked me. Their stories were exactly the same. Both of them were lies. But I still ended up in prison [on remand]. And

I remember thinking 'this ain't for me'. It broke my mother's heart when she visited me in there. I wasn't going to go back there. I got off, and I've never looked back. My place was in the club. And I've never been out of work.

The goalposts are usually, and predictably, quite fixed when rubbing up against the criminal justice and social security systems but, as I noted in *The Milltown Boys Revisited* (pp.92–94), the Boys are often impressively adept at working out how and when to 'play up', 'play the game' and 'play the system'. They are not so skilled at doing so in the context of the work place, the domestic arena, and their leisure time. Many of the Boys have paid quite a heavy price for inappropriate or unacceptable reactions in those contexts or the failure to be proactive when this might have been beneficial to them. They have often been quick to argue or physically confront, slow to apologise or make amends. They have also been slow to take opportunities that may have been actively or inadvertently presented to them, at least those on the right side of the law! Tony is, of course, the great exception to this last observation and he has benefited enormously from seizing the moment, spotting his room for manoeuvre and snapping it up, though he remains modest enough to recognise that he also had some lucky breaks and timely support:

> The big breaks I got in my life were my mum sending me to the correct school. That was the biggest break for me, given where I lived. The natural school for me to go to, where the others in the streets round me went to, was the comprehensive, which was not so far away. And instead, my mum made me walk fucking miles every day to the catholic school. So that was a massive break. And then I had one good teacher who was quite like the way I have described you when I first knew you – young and enthusiastic. Sadly, I really wasted my time at school. I bunked off too much. If I could change anything about my life, I would have turned up at school a bit more.
>
> And then I went and worked for a firm that had a good MD [Managing Director], who gave me good opportunities. But, you know, I don't want to sound big-headed, but I must have been reasonably good at what I did, to get where I did with that company. And then my current business partner – he must have seen something in me that would make this company more of a success.
>
> Don't get me wrong. Over the years, I have been offered lots of jobs. It's not all down to luck. Some of it must be. But I've worked hard all my life, *all* my life. And I've really gone the extra mile, put the extra hours in. Because most of the time I've enjoyed what I've done. That makes it easier.
>
> We were very poor growing up, *very* poor. My mum was brilliant. Another good break that I had was my mum getting rid of my dad when she did. So she brought up her two younger children – me and my brother – in a stable background, rather than an unstable background, which my older brothers and sisters had to suffer. And the two of us have both done very well for ourselves.

I don't do it often, but I'd be lying to you if I said that I've never stood here, just looking at my £600,000 house and £100,000 worth of cars on the drive and fancy holidays and all that sort of shit …

But that's just material things. Where I've been really lucky is that I've got a lovely wife, I've got beautiful kids, they've got great partners, and I've got delightful grandsons. And that's the most important thing, and not the frippery.

At the other end of the spectrum, arguably, might be Paul, who never had any self-belief that he could or would make something of his life, and who some would say 'never had a chance'.

CONCLUSION

Jamie was convinced that the striking differences in the life-course of the Boys, and particularly in relation to what he called the different 'gangs'[93] amongst the Boys, was a product of 'intelligence'. He reflected on schooling and qualifications, noting that he and most of the catholic Boys had gone to a Catholic school, got at least some 'CSE's and gone on to reasonably successful futures, unlike the "gang from up the top", who had attended the local comprehensive and largely (in fact all but Shaun[94]) left with no qualifications at all. But Jamie almost immediately had second thoughts and retracted that perspective and generalisation. After all, he acknowledged, Marty, Mack and one or two others who later came to be aligned – in terms of group membership and lifestyle – with *The Fountain* Boys (even if they didn't always drink in *The Fountain*) had attended the Catholic school, though none of them gained any qualifications. Conversely, though he too had attended the Catholic school, 'five-star Beechy' (Tony) had come from the very epicentre of deprivation and delinquency (the streets occupied by the 'gang from up the top') and yet turned out to become indisputably one of the most successful of the Boys. Perhaps more problematically, Gary – at the age of 11 possibly the hardest (alongside Ted) of the new kids at the comprehensive – also had a successful transition to adulthood, having joined up with the catholic Boys in his late teens. Nutter, however, had made the same move, but never curtailed his drinking and ended up camping in the woods.

---

93 Jamie is talking here about sub-groupings of the Boys, not 'gangs' in any formal academic or media-fuelled sense of the word.

94 Shaun's three 'CSE's (Certificate of Secondary Education) were sufficient for him to secure an apprenticeship to become an electrician. That set him on quite a different path from all the other Boys who attended the comprehensive school, none of whom achieved any educational qualifications at all.

And that is the conundrum in any effort to theorise about the Boys and to develop an argument that might plausibly be applied to a broader population of men born into very similar circumstances in 1960. Like the TV series 7 *Up*, which has followed a cohort of children from a similar period (those born in 1958) but from very *different* backgrounds, it is almost impossible to anticipate what may happen next or, looking back, to explain why particular turning points took place (or, indeed, did not). The Boys have their views, academics clearly have theirs and, in my own hybrid way, I have mine.

What is clear is that it is very unlikely that such a study could ever be done again. Class and culture are, today, more diverse, diffuse and fragmented. One would be hard-pressed to find a group of boys, even within one neighbourhood, coming from almost identical backgrounds, with very little to distinguish one from another. Though, from a sociological point of view, certainly trapped in their working-class roots, the Boys were also – perhaps paradoxically – free agents and free spirits. When they were teenagers, nobody seemed to mind what they did; nobody seemed to care. It was as if they had a licence to be carefree, unless they were incarcerated! And the Boys exercised that liberty with abandon – drinking, smoking, sniffing glue, stealing cars, fighting and shagging (I was going to write 'loving', but, with one or two exceptions, that would have been a lie). Jamie described the Boys as "sensible idiots… if you can say that?", and suggested some had more sense than others. Some learned to draw the line, to desist from offending, to get reasonable work, to 'settle down' (described as to 'go missing' in *The Milltown Boys Revisited*), in short – to grow up, though most preserved some slots within their weekly routines to 'stay young' – notably through heavy drinking on Saturday nights.

The other thing that could no longer be replicated was my approach to research. I was never covert about it (see Calvey 2017), either to the Boys, their families and their friends, or to officialdom (social workers, the police, the courts and others), or to my academic colleagues. The Boys did come to my house. I did have weekly 'gambling' sessions (you simply cannot play three-card brag without money, though you can limit the bets to coppers; no silver was ever allowed – Tommy turned up once and slapped a pocket full of silver on the table; I told him, if he wanted to play for those amounts, he should go to the pub). I introduced the Boys to *my* friends and family and colleagues. I still do. Academic colleagues and professionals often look askance when I tell them how I related to the Boys, but it was different times. Such contact and approach might well struggle to get through university ethics procedures today. At that time, there were no such procedures at all!

What did materialise from those relationships, however, was a close, unusual but rather special bond between me as a 'youth worker', researcher and 'friend', and 'the Boys', that helped me to uncover the hidden depths of their life experiences and perspectives, and to illuminate them for wider consumption. We learned from each other and, though I gleaned an encyclopaedic understanding of their milieu and *modus operandi*, there is still one regret I have: as I have noted, the Boys were habitual gamblers (on horses, dogs and football) and yet I had never once asked them – either formally in a research interview or during more casual conversations – about the detail of it. I don't know why. I still don't really understand what an 'accumulator' is, though I can hazard a guess. I have never set foot in a betting shop and today, with the proliferation of online betting, it is almost certainly now too late!

When I thanked Tony for the time he had given me to do the research interview, he said it was not a problem – the invoice was already in the post! The repartee of a lifetime has never stopped.

The last word, however, should rest with Spaceman, however much he dislikes his pseudonym. Our reunion when I was preparing for the last book was rather unexpected, but it has spawned a rather special relationship. I was even unsure that it was him as we passed each other in a busy shopping centre in 1999 (see *The Milltown Boys Revisited*, p.12). But I called out his childhood nickname that had stuck with him until today (amongst the Boys at least) and he span around. We went for a cup of tea in a nearby outdoor café, where he told me he was in the middle of his art degree. Over the years since, we have become genuine friends and shared quite a lot of time together. As he had done for *The Milltown Boys Revisited*, after considerable argument and eventually agreement, I wanted him to paint the cover of this book. We agreed that perhaps it could be a creative interpretation of a photograph taken in the 2010s of a wall in Milltown, adjacent to some wasteland where some of the Boys' own childhood homes had once stood before they were demolished, on which the 1974 graffiti by many of the Boys was still visible nearly 50 years later (with their names, nicknames and 'Slade' and, of course, 'Bowie'), and that we would change their names to those they are called in the book. I explained that although I had drawn on knowledge of the current situation of nearly all the Boys in the earlier books, I had deliberately interviewed some from each of the three broad groups identified in 2000: some of The Fountain Boys, some of the 'catholic' Boys, and some of those somewhere in the middle – those, Spaceman interjected, who had "never left home". But, as before, they are still hard to classify because there are so many overlaps, similarities and differences, between them, except perhaps at the polar extremes of the spectrum. Revealing all those nuanced crossovers in their lives is, indeed, the purpose of the book.

And it was at this point in the conversation about the cover picture that Spaceman launched into one of his valuable and informed monologues:

> When we were kids, we were in and out of each other's houses, staying over… we were like family really. I mean, I've known these guys for 55 years or whatever; it's a long time, H. It's great, although it can get boring, sometimes, well not boring but, you know, sometimes it can feel like you've said it all. But it's still wonderful. None of those are stale friendships. I mean, there's still life in all those friendships, even when you don't always see some of them so much. There's still plenty of mileage there. I mean, you go on about us being loyal to each other. Well that's what it is. Once we close in, you can't get in. Nobody can penetrate us. It's a great thing, because we can do that if we want to, even if we don't really want to do that, most of the time, because – at

the end of the day – we're nice blokes who want to get on with people. I've hardly ever had a bad argument with any of them, never fallen out. You might step back a bit, for a couple of weeks, to think about something. It's never been, you're fucking not part of us any more, fuck off. Nobody's ever been kicked out. It really is like a family, in a lot of ways much better than that!

This may be a slightly romantic interpretation of 'the Boys' but, at the same time, it is not in fact so far from the truth. I am just very appreciative that, fairly unconditionally, they let me in.

BIBLIOGRAPHY

Andrews, M. (1993), *Lifetimes of Commitment: Aging, Politics, Psychology*, Cambridge: Cambridge University Press

Ashton, D. and Field, D. (1976), *Young Workers: From School to Work*, London: Hutchinson

Atkinson, D. (1995), *Cities of Pride: Rebuilding Communities, Refocusing Government*, London: Cassell

Beck, U. (1992), *Risk Society: Towards a New Modernity*, London: Sage

Becker, H. (1963), *Outsiders: Studies in the Sociology Deviance*, New York: The Free Press

Bell, D. and Blanchflower, D. (2011), *Young People and the Great Recession*, IZA Discussion Papers No 5674, Bonn: Institute for the Study of Labor

Bukodi, E. and Goldthorpe, J. (2018), *Social Mobility and Education in Britain: Research, Politics and Policy*, Cambridge: Cambridge University Press

Calvey, D. (2017) *Covert Research: The Art, Politics and Ethics of Undercover Fieldwork*, London: Sage

Campbell, B. (1993), *Goliath: Britain's Dangerous Places*, London: Methuen

Cashmore, E. (1984), *No Future: Youth and Society*, London: Heinemann

Cloward, R. and Ohlin, L. (1960), *Delinquency and Opportunity*, London: Routledge and Kegan Paul

Cohen, P. (1997), *Rethinking the Youth Question: Education, Labour and Cultural Studies*, London: Macmillan

Cohen, S. (1972), *Folk Devils and Moral Panics*, London: Paladin

Connell, R. (1995), *Masculinities*, Cambridge: Polity Press

Connelly, F. and Clandinin, J. (2006), 'Narrative inquiry', in J. Green, G. Camilli and P. Elmore (eds), *Handbook of Complimentary Methods in Education Research* New Jersey: Lawrence Erlbaum

Davin, A. (1996), *Growing Up Poor: Home, School and Street in London 1870–1914*, London: Rivers Oram Press

Denzin, N. (1975), Review of 'The Professional Fence' by Carl Klockars, *American Journal of Sociology*, Vol 81 No 3, pp.671–673

Drakeford, M. (1997), *Social Movements and Their Supporters: The Green Shirts in England*, London: Macmillan

Emlyn-Jones, A. (2015), *A Torn Tapestry*, Cardiff: Pen-yr-Enfys Press

Evans, G. (1956), *Ask the Fellows who cut the Hay*, London: Faber and Faber

Evans, G. (1987), *Spoken History*, London: Faber and Faber

Evans, K. (1998), *Shaping Futures: Learning for Competence and Citizenship*, Aldershot: Ashgate

Evans, K. and Furlong, A. (1997), 'Metaphors of youth transitions: niches, pathways, trajectories or navigations', in J. Bynner, L. Chisholm and A. Furlong (eds), *Youth, Citizenship and Social Change in a European Context*, Aldershot: Ashgate

Giddens, A. (1991), *Modernity and Self-Identity: Self and Society in a Late Modern Age*, Oxford: Polity Press

Giddens, A. (1998), *The Third Way: The Renewal of Democracy*, Cambridge: Polity Press

Gittens, D. (1979), 'Oral history: reliability and recollection', in L. Moss and H. Goldstein (eds), *The Recall Method in Social Surveys*, London: Institute of Education

Glueck, S. and Glueck, E. (1950), *Unraveling Juvenile Delinquency*, New York: Commonwealth Fund

Goldthorpe, J. Lockwood, D., Bechofer, F. and Platt, J. (1969), *The Affluent Worker*, London: Cambridge University Press

Griffiths, G. (1989), 'Museums and the Practice of Oral History', *Journal of Oral History*, Autumn, pp.49–51

Hall, S. and Jefferson, T. (eds) (1976), *Resistance through Rituals*, London: Hutchinson

Halsey, A. H. (1996), *No Discouragement*, London: Macmillan

Halsey, A. H., Heath, A. and Ridge, J. (1980), *Origins and Destinations: Family, Class and Education in Modern Britain*, Oxford: Clarendon Press

Hayman, J. (2017), *British Journey*, Kibworth Beauchamp: Matador

Helve, H. and Bynner, J. (eds) (1996), *Youth and Life Management: Research Perspectives*, Helsinki: Helsinki University Press

Herbert, D. and Evans, D. (1974), *Urban Environment and Juvenile Delinquency*, Home Office Report, Swansea University: Department of Geography

Holland, J. (2007), 'Emotions and research', *International Journal of Social Research Methodology*, Vol 10 No 3, pp.195–209

Hooley, T. (2009), *Adventures in Career Development: The Milltown Boys Revisited*, Wordpress October 14

Istance, D., Rees, G. and Williamson, H. (1994), *Young People Not in Education, Training or Employment in South Glamorgan*, Cardiff: South Glamorgan Training and Enterprise Council

Jones, P., Williamson, H., Payne, J. and Smith, G. (1982), *Out of School: A Case Study of the Role of Government Schemes at a Time of Growing Unemployment*, London: Manpower Services Commission

Klockars, C. (1975), *The Professional Fence*, London: Tavistock

Laub, J. and Sampson, R. (2003), *Shared Beginnings, Divergent Lives: Delinquent Boys to Age 70*, Cambridge, Mass: Harvard University Press

Lee, G. and Wrench, J. (1983), *Skill Seekers – Black Youth, Apprenticeships and Disadvantage*, Leicester: National Youth Bureau

Lemert, E. (1951), *Social Pathology*, New York: Mcgraw Hill

Lieberman, A. and Tobin, B. (1983), *The Experience of Old Age: Stress, Coping and Survival*, New York: Basic Books

Loughran, T. and Mannay, D. (2018), 'Introduction: why emotion matters', in T. Loughran and D. Mannay (eds), *Emotion and the Researcher: Sites, Subjectivities and Relationships*, Studies in Qualitative Methodology Volume 16, Bingley: Emerald Publishing

Mahoney, D. (2007), 'Constructing reflexive fieldwork relationships: narrating my collaborative storytelling methodology', *Qualitative Inquiry*, Vol 13 No 4, pp.573–594

Manpower Services Commission (1976), *Instructional Guide to Social and Life Skills Training*, London: Manpower Services Commission

Mars, G. (1982), *Cheats at Work: A Social Anthropology of Workplace Crime*, London: Allen & Unwin

Martin, H. (2020), *The Reacher Guy*, New York: Little Brown

Matza, D. (1964), *Delinquency and Drift*, New York: Wiley

Ministry of Justice/HM Prison and Probation Service (2020), *Home Detention Curfew (HDC) Policy Framework*, London: Ministry of Justice

Mungham, G. and Pearson, G. (1976), *Working Class Youth Culture*, London: Routledge and Kegan Paul

Parker, H. (1974), *View from the Boys: A Sociology of Downtown Adolescents*, Newton Abbott: David and Charles

Patrick, J. (1973), *A Glasgow Gang Observed*, London: Methuen

Pearson, G. (1993), 'Foreword', in D. Hobbs and T. May (eds), *Interpreting the Field: Accounts of Ethnography*, Oxford: Oxford University Press

Pharoah, N. (1963), 'The Long Blunt Shock', *New Society*, 26 September

Pilcher, J. (1998), *Women of their Time: Generation, Gender Issues and Feminism*, Aldershot: Ashgate

Public Health Wales NHS Trust (2015), *Adverse Childhood Experiences and their Impact on Health-Harming Behaviours in the Welsh Adult Population*, Cardiff: Public Health Wales

Putnam, R. (2000), *Bowling Alone: The Collapse and Revival of American Community*, New York: Simon and Schuster

Sampson, R. and Laub, J. (1995), *Crime in the Making: Pathways and Turning Points through Life*, Cambridge, Mass: Harvard University Press

Social Exclusion Unit (1999), *Bridging the Gap: New Opportunities for Young People Not in Education, Employment or Training*, London: The Stationery Office

Social Exclusion Unit (2000), *National Strategy for Neighbourhood Renewal: Report of Policy Action Team 12 – Young People*, London: The Stationery Office

Spradley, J. (1979), *The Ethnographic Interview*, New York: Holt, Rinhart Winston

Standing, G. (2011), *The Precariat: The New Dangerous Class*, London: Bloomsbury

Swartz, S. (2021), 'Navigational capacities for Southern youth in adverse contexts' in S. Swartz, A. Cooper, C. Batan and L. Kropff Causa (eds), *The Oxford Handbook of Global South Youth Studies*, New York: Oxford University Press

Swartz, S. and Cooper, A. (2014), *Navigational capacities for youth success in adversity: a sociology of southern youth*, paper presented at the XVIII World Congress of Sociology, Yokohama, Japan

Sykes, G. and Matza, D. (1957), 'Techniques of neutralisation: a theory of delinquency', *American Sociological Review* Vol 22, pp.664–670

Terkel, S. (1970), *Hard Times: An Illustrated Oral History of the Great Depression*, New York: Pantheon Books

Terkel, S. (1974), *Working: People Talk About What They Do All Day and How They Feel About What They Do*, New York: Pantheon Books

Terkel, S. (2003), *Hope Dies Last: Keeping the Faith in Difficult Times*, New York: The New Press

The Health Foundation (2020), *Health Equity in England: The Marmot Review 10 years on)*, London: The Health Foundation

Thomas, H. (1979), *The Spanish Civil War*, Harmondsworth: Penguin

Thompson, P. (1978), *The Voice of the Past*, Oxford: Oxford University Press

Treadwell, J. (2020), *Criminological Ethnography: An Introduction*, London: Sage

Tristram, G. (2014), *JB's: The Story of Dudley's Legendary Live Music Venue*, Stourbridge: The Drawing Room Press

Webbe, G. (2019), *The Gloves Are Off*, Talybont: Y Lolfa Cyf

Whyte, W. (1943), *Street Corner Society: The Social Structure of an Italian Slum*, Chicago: University of Chicago Press

Williams, G. (2017), *Ask the Fellows who Cut the Coal: George Ewart Evans of Abercynon 1909– 1988*, Pontypridd: Keelin

Williamson, H. (1978), 'Choosing to be a delinquent', *New Society* 9 November

Williamson, H. (1981), *Juvenile Justice and the Working-Class Community*, unpublished PhD thesis

Williamson, H. (1987), *Toolmaking and Politics: The Life of Ted Smallbone – An Oral History*, Birmingham: Linden Books

Williamson, H. (1996), 'Systematic or Sentimental? The place of feelings in social research', in K. Carter and S. Delamont (eds), *Qualitative Research: The Emotional Dimension*, Aldershot: Avebury

Williamson, H. (1997), '"Status Zer0" and the "underclass": some considerations', in R. MacDonald (ed.), *Youth, the 'Underclass' and Social Exclusion*, London: Routledge

Williamson, H. (2004a), *The Milltown Boys Revisited*, Oxford: Berg

Williamson, H. (2004b), 'Young people can say the funniest things', *Young People Now* 12–18 May, p.15

Williamson, H. (2012), *Eggs in a Pan – The Emergence of Youth Policy in Europe*, Pontypridd: University of Glamorgan

Williamson, H. (2017), 'Winning space, building bridges – what youth work is all about', in H. Schild, N. Connolly, F. Labadie, J. Vanhee and H. Williamson (eds), *Thinking Seriously About Youth Work*, Strasbourg: Council of Europe

Williamson, H. (2014), 'Stories of "lifetime NEETs" will often end in tragedy', *Children and Young People Now*, 29 April–12 May, p.21

Williamson, H. (2021), '*There's Always Tomorrow* - Strengthening agency and challenging structure through youth work and youth policy', in A. Caetano and M. Nico (eds), *Structure and Agency in Young People's Lives: Theory, Methods and Agendas*, London: Routledge

Williamson, H. and Weatherspoon, K. (1985), *Strategies for Intervention: An Approach to Youth and Community Work in an Area of Social Deprivation*, Cardiff: University College Cardiff Social Research Unit

Williamson, H. and Williamson, P. (1981), *Five Years*, Leicester: National Youth Bureau

Willis, P. (1978), *Learning to Labour: How Working-Class Kids Get Working-Class Jobs*, Farnborough: Saxon House

Wilson, A. (2007), *Northern Soul: Music, Drugs and Subcultural Identity*, Cullompton: Willan

Wright Mills, C. (1970), *The Sociological Imagination*, Harmondsworth: Penguin

Young, J. (1971), *The Drugtakers: The Social Meaning of Drug Use*, London: Paladin

Young, M. (1958), *The Rise of the Meritocracy*, London: Thames and Hudson

INDEX